Psychology of Voice Disorders

Psychology of Voice Disorders

Deborah Caputo Rosen, R.N., Ph.D.

Medical Psychologist
Otolaryngologic Nurse-Clinician

Research Associate
American Institute for Voice and Ear Research

Consulting Psychologist
Dept. of Otolaryngology—Head and Neck Surgery
The Graduate Hospital
Philadelphia, Pennsylvania

Robert Thayer Sataloff, M.D., D.M.A.

Professor of Otolaryngology
Thomas Jefferson University

Chairman
Department of Otolaryngology—Head and Neck Surgery
The Graduate Hospital

Adjunct Professor of Otorhinolaryngology—Head and Neck Surgery
University of Pennsylvania
Philadelphia, Pennsylvania

Adjunct Professor of Otolaryngology—Head and Neck Surgery
Georgetown University
Washington, D.C.

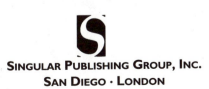

SINGULAR PUBLISHING GROUP, INC.
SAN DIEGO · LONDON

Singular Publishing Group, Inc.
401 West A Street, Suite 325
San Diego, California 92101-7904

19 Compton Terrace
London N1 2UN, U.K.

e-mail: singpub@mail.cerfnet.com
Website: http://www.singpub.com

Typeset in 10/12 Palatino by So Cal Graphics
Printed in the United States of America by McNaughton & Gunn

Library of Congress Cataloging-in-Publication Data

Rosen, Deborah Caputo.
    Psychology of voice disorders / Deborah Caputo Rosen, Robert
Thayer Sataloff.
       p.   cm.
    Includes bibliographical references and index.
    ISBN 1-56593-839-9
    1. Voice disorders—Psychological aspects. 2. Voice disorders—
Patients—Rehabilitation. I. Sataloff, Robert Thayer. II. Title.
    [DNLM: 1. Voice Disorders—psychology.   WV 500 R813p 1997]
RF510.R67   1997
616.85'5'0019—dc21
DNLM/DLC
for Library of Congress   96-50038
                                                     CIP

CONTENTS

PREFACE

This book is intended as a text to guide mental health professionals called on to care for patients with voice disorders. The voice is extremely important to many people, and the psychological concomitants of voice disorders may be profound, especially in professional voice users. This population used to be thought of as limited to singers, actors and a few other professionals. However, it is now clear that many other people use their voices professionally and may have a great deal of their self-concept, self-esteem, and personality invested in vocal quality, health, and endurance. It is essential for psychological professionals to understand the special psychological impact of disorders of the voice. The terms psychological professional and psychotherapist are used throughout the text to refer to caregivers from any of the mental health disciplines, including psychiatrists, psychologists, clinical social workers, psychiatric nurse clinical specialists, and mental health counselors. The term arts medicine medical psychologist is applied to any psychological professional with advanced clinical training in these fields of subspecialization.

In order to manage psychological problems in voice patients expertly, clinicians must be knowledgeable about many aspects of voice care provided by other disciplines. This book is intended to discuss in an introductory fashion many of the medical subjects with which psychological professionals should be familiar. However, interested readers are encouraged to consult other sources[1,2] for more information and to affiliate with a medical voice care team to acquire practical knowledge and insights.

In addition to providing an introduction to relevant medical management of voice patients, current theories on the etiology and major identifying features of common voice-related psychological problems are presented in detail, some for the first time. Treatment strategies that have proven efficacious are described. Because this is the first textbook on this interdisciplinary subject, omissions and shortcomings will become apparent over the next few years, and ongoing research by arts medicine and other health psychology specialists will offer contributions which extend clinical practice. The book is offered at this time in an effort to share extensive clinical experience and to encourage further investigation.

In our medical practice, we see approximately 1200 professional voice visits annually; and psychological factors are important to some degree in nearly all of them. A minority of those patients require formal psychological therapy; but without evaluation that is sensitive to potential emotional impact, most would go unrecognized and untreated. Unfortunately, this is the case in most medical centers; and even when patients with psychological problems are recognized and referred for therapy, too often they are treated by therapists without expertise in special voice-related issues.

This book attempts to systematically provide therapists with the special knowledge they need. Although it is directed primarily at psychotherapists, it is also intended to be useful for voice therapists, nurse-specialists, and laryngologists. The introductory chapter provides an overview of the field of voice and highlights the interdisciplinary nature of voice care. Chapter 2 reviews in accessible language the modern concepts of voice analysis and physiology, introducing terminology the therapist will need to communicate with other colleagues on the voice treatment team. Chapter 3 explains the medical history and physical examination, pointing out the need for psychotherapists to understand clearly the patient's medical diagnosis and prognosis. Chapter 4 discusses many common diagnoses and treatments, illustrating the importance to voice performance of many systemic disorders distant from the head and neck. Chapter 5 provides a comprehensive discussion of many common medications that may affect voice performance, emphasizing the side effects associated with psychotropic medications. Chapter 6 presents principles of psychological assessment for patients with voice disorders. The chapter provides specific details, recommendations, and philosophies regarding the approach to this patient population. It also discusses special considerations that arise from the psychologist's collaboration with a medical-model voice care team. Special psychological problems arising in professional voice users are introduced.

Chapter 7 discusses co-morbid psychopathology found in a population of professional voice users, and the implications of these conditions for voice performance. Chapter 8 reveals the factors that underlie special psychological problems that result from voice disturbance in professional voice users, highlighting personality type and self-esteem issues and their consequences. Chapter 9 addresses the complex subject of psychogenic dysphonia. Psychological reactions are seen routinely among patients with voice disorders, but occasionally voice disorders are caused primarily by psychological factors. In addition to presenting these factors, insights are provided on how to differentiate psychogenic from organic voice disturbance, and how to treat psychogenic dysphonia.

Chapters 10 and 11 are particularly important and unique. Recognizing the importance of a professional's voice to his or her identity and self-esteem, these chapters explain the emotional responses to vocal fold injury or surgery. The phases of reaction to vocal fold injury or surgery are detailed. Information is provided that explains the often extreme psychological reactions to vocal injury, predicts the course of psychological response, and guides the therapy. Guidelines are also given for counseling approaches which help avoid or minimize troubling responses for many patients. Chapter 12 reviews the many neurological disorders that may be accompanied by voice, speech, or language disturbance. Some of these neurological conditions are known to be accompanied by psychological changes caused by the underlying neurologic process. In others, psychological reactions are secondary to impairment of verbal communication ability. This chapter addresses both situations and includes guidelines to differentiate and treat psychological factors. Vocal tract cancer results in profound psychological disturbance in many patients. This is caused by impairment (or perceived threatened impairment) of verbal communication, abrupt change in self-image and esteem (as may follow laryngectomy), and the issues of having cancer. Special problems associated with vocal tract cancers in voice professionals are emphasized.

Stress is a major problem for voice professionals, whether they are singers, actors, politicians, clergy, teachers, public speakers, or others. Chapter 14 discusses techniques for managing stress in voice patients in general, and in the professional population, in particular. Performance anxiety is a special form of stress. It is discussed in detail in Chapter 15. Chapter 16 discusses psychotherapeutic management of the voice disordered patient in detail. This lengthy chapter lays out the principles for managing psychological problems in patients with voice disorders. Chapter 17 enhances Chapter 16 by presenting in detail previously unpublished insights into the principles of psychological dysfunction and treatment in voice professionals and providing detailed case studies to illustrate treatment techniques. These are enhanced by the use of art as an analytic and treatment instrument. The appendices include in their entirety the questionnaires, history forms, and instruments referred to in the text.

It is our hope that this text will improve therapists' insight and treatment in this patient population and also inspire additional research that advances this young and vital subspecialty of psychological care.

Deborah Caputo Rosen, R.N., Ph.D.
Robert Thayer Sataloff, M.D., D.M.A.

REFERENCES

1. Sataloff RT: *Professional Voice: Science and Art of Clinical Care,* 2nd ed. San Diego, Calif: Singular Publishing Group Inc; 1997.
2. Sataloff RT. The human voice, *Sci Am.* 1992;267(6):108-115.

ACKNOWLEDGMENTS

From DCR:

To my parents, Edward and Carolyn Caputo, who gave me ROOTS: my "love for beautiful language" and "Sunday morning music"; and all those who gave me WINGS: Alyssa and Jacob Rosen, who thrived so magnificently on my energy leftovers; my colleagues Bob Sataloff, Joe Spiegel, Mary Hawkshaw, Bud Heuer, Peggy Baroody, Kate Emerich, Rhonda Rulnick, Cheryl Hoover, Caren Sokolow, Debra Levin and Maestro Harold Evans, who gave so generously of their knowledge and humanity; to Lori Maccarone, Linda Pizzo, and Maria Lampe, who insisted I remember how to keep a playful spirit in my work; to Jonathan Oehler, my transcriptionist, grammarian, and friend, whose assistance was invaluable in the preparation of this manuscript; and to Cathy and Michael Frank, who nourished my body, mind, and spirit throughout the writing of this book. My grateful thanks

From RTS:

This book could not have been written without years of dedicated collaboration among all the members of our office staff, and our patients. We are indebted to all who worked with us as the concepts in this book evolved and who helped us articulate them. Special thanks go to my family who tolerate so many evenings and vacations spent with a dictaphone.

About the Authors

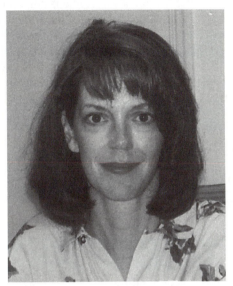

Deborah Caputo, Rosen, R.N., Ph.D.

Deborah Caputo Rosen is a licensed clinical psychologist specializing in medical psychology. She is also a certified otolaryngologic nurse clinician in association with Drs. Joseph Sataloff, Robert T. Sataloff, and Joseph Spiegel in Philadelphia, Pennsylvania. She maintains a private practice in psychology and clinical hypnosis specializing in the psychological impact of communication disorders and grief and loss issues. Dr. Rosen is the Research Associate of the American Institute for Voice and Ear Research. She received her Diploma in Nursing from the Lankenau Hospital School of Nursing, her Bachelor of Science in Sociology with a concentration in community health from St. Joseph's University, her Master of Science in Counseling and Human Relations from Villanova University, and her doctorate in Clinical Psychology from the Union Institute Graduate School.

In addition to her licensure as a registered nurse and clinical psychologist, she is also a certified practitioner of Ericksonian hypnosis and Neurolinguistic Programming and a Certified Professional Grief Counsellor. Dr. Rosen is a consulting psychologist at The Graduate Hospital in the Department of Otolaryngology—Head and Neck Surgery. She is a member of the Association for Death Education and

Counseling, the American Association for Counseling and Development, and the American Mental Health Counselors' Association. Dr. Rosen serves on the Board of Directors for The Voice Foundation and the Editorial Board of the *Journal of Voice*. She is currently the President of the Southeastern Pennsylvania Chapter of the Society of Otolaryngologic and Head and Neck Nurses (SOHN). She has authored or co-authored numerous book chapters and journal articles. Dr. Rosen is a frequent presenter of seminars, lectures, and courses on psychological components of health maintenance, communication disorders, and grief and loss issues.

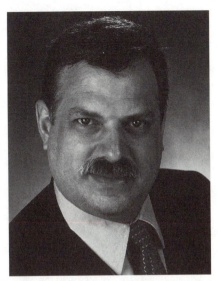

Robert Thayer Sataloff, M.D., D.M.A.

Robert T. Sataloff, M.D., D.M.A. is Professor of Otolaryngology at Jefferson Medical College, Thomas Jefferson University, and Chairman of the Department of Otolaryngology—Head and Neck Surgery at the Graduate Hospital (in affiliation with the University of Pennsylvania), Adjunct Associate Professor of Otorhinolaryngology—Head and Neck Surgery, the University of Pennsylvania, Adjunct Professor of Otolaryngology—Head and Neck Surgery at Georgetown University, on the Faculties of the Academy of Vocal Arts and the Curtis Institute of Music, Conductor of the Thomas Jefferson University Choir and Orchestra, Director of the Jefferson Arts-Medicine Center, and Chairman of the Boards of Directors of the Voice Foundation and of the American Institute for Voice and Ear Research. Dr. Sataloff is also a professional singer and singing teacher. He holds an undergraduate degree from Haverford College in Music Theory and Composition, graduated from Jefferson Medical College, received a Doctor of Musical Arts in Voice Performance from Combs College of Music, and completed his Residency in Otolaryngology—Head and Neck Surgery at the University of Michigan. He also completed a Fellowship in Otology, Neurotology and Skull Base Surgery at the University of Michigan. He is Editor-in-Chief of the *Journal of Voice*, on the Editorial Board of the *Journal of Singing*, *Medical Problems of Performing Artists*, and *Ear, Nose & Throat Journal*, and on the Editorial Review Boards of most major otolaryngology journals in the United States. Dr. Sataloff has written over 400 publications, including 13 textbooks. His medical practice is limited to care of the professional voice and to neurotology—skull base surgery. Dr. Sataloff's books include:

Sataloff J, Sataloff RT, Vassallo LA. *Hearing Loss.* Philadelphia, Penna: JB Lippincott; 1980.

Sataloff, RT, Sataloff J. *Occupational Hearing Loss.* New York, NY: Marcel Dekker; 1987.

Sataloff, RT, Brandfonbrener A, Lederman R. *Textbook of Performing Arts Medicine.* New York, NY: Raven Press; 1991.

Sataloff, RT. *Embryology and Anomalies of the Facial Nerve.* New York, NY: Raven Press; 1991.

Sataloff RT. *Professional Voice: The Science and Art of Clinical Care,* New York, NY: Raven Press; 1991.

Sataloff, RT, Titze IR. *Vocal Health and Science.* The National Association of Teachers of Singing, Jacksonville, Florida, 1991.

Gould, WJ, Sataloff RT, Spiegel JR. *Voice Surgery.* St. Louis, MO.: CV Mosby Co; 1993.

Sataloff RT, Sataloff J. *Occupational Hearing Loss* 2nd ed. NY, NY: Marcel Dekker; 1993.

Mandel S, Sataloff RT, Schapiro S. *Minor Head Trauma: Assessment, Management and Rehabilitation.* New York, NY: Springer-Verlag; 1993.

Sataloff RT, Sataloff J. *Hearing Loss* 3rd ed. New York, NY: Marcel Dekker; 1993.

Rubin J, Sataloff RT, Korovin G, Gould WJ. *The Diagnosis and Treatment of Voice Disorders.* New York, NY; Igaku-Shoin Medical Publishers, Inc, 1995.

Rosen DC, Sataloff RT. *The Psychology of Voice Disorders.* San Diego, CA: Singular Publishing Group, Inc; In press.

CHAPTER

1

Introduction

"Voice" is the newest subspecialty of otolaryngology. It evolved as an outgrowth of interest in the problems of professional singers and actors.[1] Voice medicine and hand medicine led the way for the development of Arts Medicine, a multispecialty discipline dedicated to the care of performers and other artists.[2] As Arts Medicine in general and voice medicine in particular have evolved, healthcare providers have learned a great deal from their involvement with performing artists.

Professional performers are not only demanding, but also remarkably self-analytical. Like athletes, performers have forced healthcare providers to change our definition of normalcy. Ordinarily, physicians, psychotherapists, and other professionals are granted great latitude in the definition of "normal." For example, if a microsurgeon injures his or her finger, and the hand surgeon restores 95% of function, the surgeon-patient is likely to be satisfied. If the same result occurs in a world class violinist, that last 5% (or 1%) may mean the difference between renown and obscurity. Traditionally, we have not been trained to recognize, let alone quantify and restore, these degrees of physical perfection. Arts medicine practitioners have learned to do so, especially in the field of voice. The process has required advances in scientific knowledge, clinical management, technology for voice assessment, voice therapy, methodology, and surgical technique. The drive to expand our knowledge has also led to unprecedented teamwork and interdisciplinary collaboration. As a result, voice care professionals have come to recognize important psychological problems commonly found in patients with voice disorders. Such problems were routinely ignored in past years. Now they are sought for diligently throughout evaluation and treatment. When identified, they often require intervention by a psychological professional who is as specialized and knowledgeable as other members of the voice care team.

Arts Medicine psychologists specializing in management of performance anxiety are becoming more common; but there are still very few psychological professionals with extensive experience in diagnosing and treating other psychological concomitants of voice disorders. The information in this book has evolved over the course of several years of close collaboration among voice team members including laryngologists, psychological professionals, nurses, speech-language pathologists, singing voice specialists, acting voice trainers, and others. The insights and recommendations contained here have evolved from extensive clinical experience with professional voice users and other voice patients, experience with general psychotherapeutic practice, and applied clinical research. The insights we have gained regarding psychological problems associated with voice disorders apply not only to voice professionals, but to nearly all voice patients.

The first task in treating any patient with a voice complaint is to establish an accurate diagnosis. This responsibility falls largely on the laryngologist. Diagnosis is achieved through a thorough, comprehensive history and physical examination, objective testing, assessment by other voice team members, and specialized examination.[3] It is essential for psychological professionals working with voice disordered patients to be familiar with this process and to understand the nature and implications of organic voice disorders. Clarification of organic dysfunction and medical prognosis is essential in the psychological management of these patients. Psychological responses in voice patients frequently do not seem initially to be proportional to the severity of voice complaints. In some people, even minor voice injuries or health problems can be very disturbing; and seemingly trivial problems can be devastating to some professional voice users. In some cases, they even trigger responses that delay return of normal voice. Stress, and fear of the evaluation procedures, often heighten the problem and may distort diagnostic assessment. Moreover, some voice disorders may be entirely psychogenic, necessitating professional psychological assessment as an essential component of the diagnostic evaluation.

Patients seeking medical care for voice disorders come from the general population. Consequently, a normal distribution of co-morbid psychopathology can be expected in a laryngology practice. Psychological factors can be causally related to a voice disorder and/or consequences of the vocal dysfunction. They are usually interwoven. The essential role of the voice in communication of the "self" creates special potential for psychological impact. Severe psychological consequences of voice dysfunction are especially common in individuals in whom the voice is pathologically perceived to be the "self," such as professional singers. However, the sensitive clinician will recognize varying degrees of similar reaction among most voice patients who are confronted with voice change or loss.

In all human beings, self-esteem is comprised not only of who we believe we are, but also what we believe we do. A psychological "double-exposure" exists for performers who experience difficulty in separating those two elements. The voice is in, is therefore of, indeed *is* the self. Aronson's[4] extensive review of the literature provides an opportunity to examine research which supports the maxim that the voice is the mirror of the personality, both normal and abnormal. Parameters such as voice quality, pitch, loudness, stress patterns, rate, pauses, articulation, vocabulary, syntax, and content are described as they reflect life stressors, psychopathology, and discrete emotions. Sundberg describes the research of Fonagy[5] on the effects of various states of emotion on phonation. These studies revealed specific alterations in articulatory and laryngeal structures and in respiratory muscular activity patterns related to 10 different emotional states. Vogel and Carter[6] include descriptive summaries of the features, symptoms, and signs of communication impairment in their text on neurologic and psychiatric disorders. The mind and body are inextricably linked. Thoughts and feelings generate neurochemical transmissions which affect all organ systems. Therefore, not only can disturbances of body function have profound emotional effects, but disturbances of emotion can have profound bodily, vocal, and artistic effects.

The following chapters are designed to supply psychological professionals with the specialized background necessary to provide optimal treatment for professional voice users and all patients with maladaptive psychological responses to vocal dysfunction. They also offer information that should enhance interaction with laryngologists, speech-language pathologists, and other professionals involved with the patient's treatment. Psychotherapists interested in working with voice disordered patients are encouraged to arrange an internship in the medical office of a laryngologist specializing in voice disorders. The insights gained in working with physicians, speech-language pathologists, singing teachers, and others in a center specializing in the care of voice patients are invaluable. Practically, this is not always possible; and this text is intended to disseminate the experience and clearly discuss the therapeutic approaches and recommendations that have arisen from our collaboration in one of the most active voice care centers.

However, no book is a substitute for clinical observation, interdisciplinary teamwork, and patient contact. Psychological professionals who are seriously interested in pursuing this fascinating, specialized area are strongly encouraged to create a collaborative opportunity of supervised practice working with an active voice team.

REFERENCES

1. Sataloff, RT. Professional singers: the science and art of clinical care. *Am J Otolaryngol.* 1981;2(3):251-266.
2. Sataloff RT, Brandfonbrener A, Lederman R. *Textbook of Performing Arts-Medicine.* New York, NY: Raven Press; 1992.
3. Sataloff RT. *Professional Voice: The Science and Art of Clinical Care,* 2nd ed. San Diego, Calif: Singular Publishing Group Inc; 1997.
4. Aronson A. *Clinical Voice Disorders,* 3rd ed. New York, NY: Thieme Medical Publishers; 1990:117-145.
5. Sundberg J. *The Science of the Singing Voice.* DeKalb, Ill: Northern Illinois University Press; 1985:146-156.
6. Vogel D, Carter J. *The Effects of Drugs on Communication Disorders.* San Diego, Calif: Singular Publishing Group Inc; 1995:31-143.

CHAPTER

2

Anatomy and Physiology of the Voice

To treat voice patients knowledgeably and responsibly, psychology professionals must understand the medical aspects of voice disorders and their treatment. This requires knowledge of the anatomy and physiology of phonation. The human voice consists of much more than simply the vocal folds, popularly known as the vocal cords. State-of-the-art voice diagnosis, nonsurgical therapy, and voice surgery depend on understanding the complex workings of the vocal tract. Psychotherapists specializing in the care of voice patients, especially voice professionals, should be familiar with at least the basics of the latest concepts in voice function. The physiology of phonation is much more complex than this brief chapter might suggest, and readers interested in acquiring more than a clinically essential introduction are encouraged to consult other literature.[1-3]

ANATOMY

The *larynx* is essential to normal voice production, but the anatomy of the voice is not limited to the larynx. The vocal mechanism includes the abdominal and back musculature, rib cage, lungs, and the pharynx, oral cavity, and nose. Each component performs an important function in voice production, although it is possible to produce voice even without a larynx, for example, in patients who have undergone laryngectomy. In addition, virtually all parts of the body play some role in voice production and may be responsible for voice dysfunction. Even something as remote as a sprained ankle may alter posture, thereby impairing abdominal, back, and thoracic muscle function and resulting in vocal inefficiency, weakness, and hoarseness.

The larynx is composed of four basic anatomic units: skeleton, intrinsic muscles, extrinsic muscles, and mucosa. The most important parts of the laryngeal skeleton are the thyroid cartilage, cricoid cartilage, and two arytenoid cartilages (Fig 2-1). Intrinsic muscles of the larynx are connected to these cartilages (Fig 2-2). One of the intrinsic muscles, the *thyroarytenoid* or *vocalis muscle*, extends on each side from the arytenoid cartilage to the inside of the thyroid cartilage just below and behind the thyroid prominence ("Adam's apple"), forming the body of the vocal folds. The vocal folds act as the *oscillator* or *voice source* of the vocal tract. The space between the vocal folds is called the *glottis* and is used as an anatomic reference point. The intrinsic muscles alter the position, shape, and tension of the vocal folds, bringing them together (adduction), moving them apart (abduction), or stretching them by increasing longitudinal tension (Fig 2-3). They are able to do so because the laryngeal cartilages are connected by soft attachments that allow changes in their relative angles and distances, thereby permitting alteration in the shape and tension of the tissues suspended between them. The arytenoid cartilages are also capable of rocking, rotating, and gliding, permitting complex vocal fold motion and alteration in the shape of the vocal fold edge (Fig 2-4). All but one of the muscles on each side of the larynx are innervated by one of the two *recurrent laryngeal nerves*. Because this nerve runs in a long course from the neck down into the chest and then back up to the larynx (hence, the name "recurrent"), it is easily injured by trauma, neck surgery, and chest surgery, which may result in vocal fold paralysis. The remaining muscle (*cricothyroid muscle*) is innervated by the superior laryngeal nerve on each side which is especially susceptible to viral and traumatic injury. It produces increases in longitudinal tension that are important in volume and pitch control. The "false vocal folds" are located above the vocal folds, and unlike the true vocal folds, usually do not make contact during normal speaking or singing.[3] The neuroanatomy and neurophysiology of phonation are extremely complicated, and only partially understood. As the new field of neurolaryngology advances, a more thorough understanding of the subject will become increasingly important to medical and psychological clinicians. Readers interested in acquiring a deeper, scientific understanding of neurophysiology are encouraged to consult the

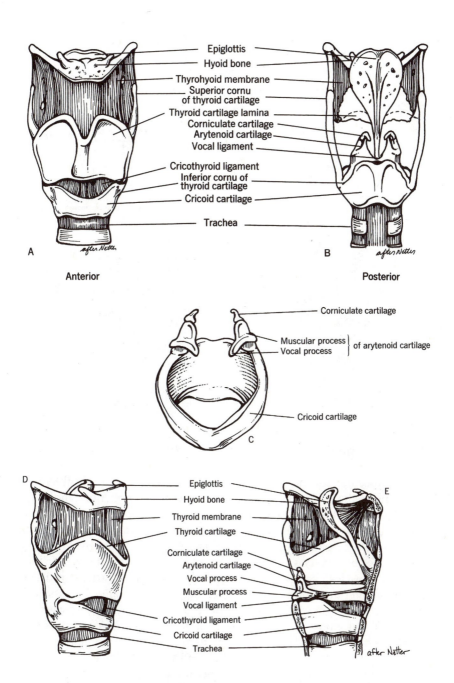

Epiglottis
Hyoid bone
Thyrohyoid membrane
Superior cornu of thyroid cartilage
Thyroid cartilage lamina
Corniculate cartilage
Arytenoid cartilage
Vocal ligament
Cricothyroid ligament
Inferior cornu of thyroid cartilage
Cricoid cartilage
Trachea

A

Anterior

B

Posterior

Corniculate cartilage
Muscular process
Vocal process } of arytenoid cartilage
Cricoid cartilage

C

D

Epiglottis
Hyoid bone
Thyroid membrane
Thyroid cartilage
Corniculate cartilage
Arytenoid cartilage
Vocal process
Muscular process
Vocal ligament
Cricothyroid ligament
Cricoid cartilage
Trachea

E

FIGURE 2-1. Cartilages of the larynx.

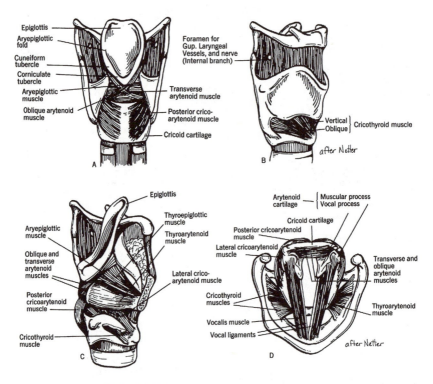

FIGURE 2-2. Intrinsic muscles of the larynx.

growing literature on this subject, particularly a well referenced review by Garrett and Larson.[4]

Because the attachments of the laryngeal cartilages are flexible, the positions of the cartilages with respect to each other change when the laryngeal skeleton is elevated or lowered. Such changes in vertical height are controlled by the extrinsic laryngeal muscles, the strap muscles of the neck. When the angles and distances between cartilages change because of this accordionlike effect, the resting length of the intrinsic muscles changes. Such large adjustments in intrinsic muscle condition interfere with fine control of smooth vocal quality.[3] Classically trained singers generally are taught to use the extrinsic muscles to maintain the laryngeal skeleton at a relatively constant height, regardless of pitch. That is, they learn to avoid the natural tendency of the larynx to rise with ascending pitch and fall with descending pitch, thereby enhancing unity of sound quality throughout the vocal range.

The soft tissues lining the larynx are much more complex than originally thought. The mucosa forms the thin, lubricated surface of the

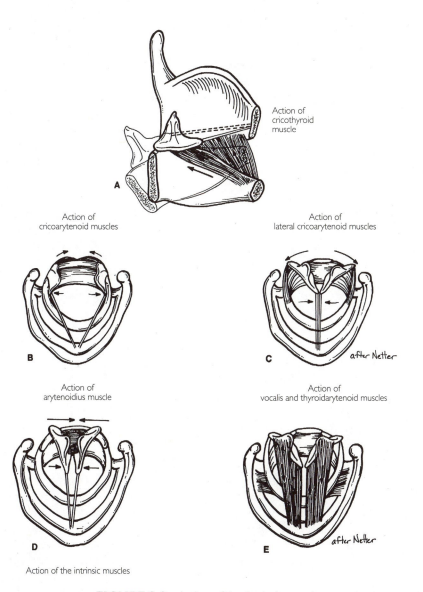

Action of
cricothyroid
muscle

Action of
cricoarytenoid muscles

Action of
lateral cricoarytenoid muscles

A

B

C

after Netter

Action of
arytenoidius muscle

Action of
vocalis and thyroidarytenoid muscles

D

E

after Netter

Action of the intrinsic muscles

FIGURE 2-3. Action of the intrinsic muscles.

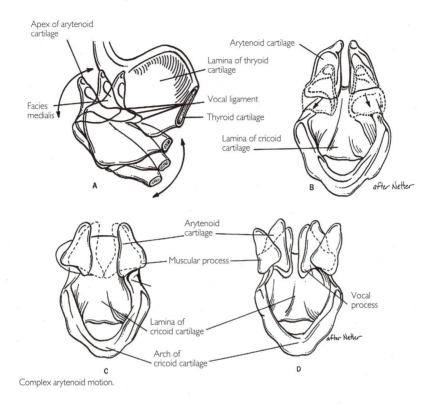

Apex of arytenoid
cartilage

Aryenoid cartilage

Lamina of thryoid
cartilage

Facies
medialis

Vocal ligament

Thyroid cartilage

Lamina of cricoid
cartilage

A   B   *after Netter*

Arytenoid
cartilage

Muscular process

Vocal
process

Lamina of
cricoid cartilage

Arch of
cricoid cartilage

C   D   *after Netter*

Complex arytenoid motion.

FIGURE 2-4. Complex arytenoid motion.

vocal folds which makes contact when the two vocal folds are approximated. Laryngeal mucosa looks superficially like the mucosa which lines the inside of the mouth. Throughout most of the larynx, there are goblet cells and pseudo-stratified ciliated columnar epithelial cells designed for handling mucous secretions, similar to mucosal surfaces found throughout the respiratory tract. However, the mucosa overlying the vocal folds is different. First, it is stratified squamous epithelium, which is better suited to withstand the trauma of vocal fold contact. Second, the vocal fold is not simply muscle covered with mucosa. Rather, it consists of five layers as described by Hirano.[5] Mechanically, the vocal fold structures act more like three layers consisting of the *cover* (epithelium and superficial layer of the lamina propria), *transition* (intermediate and deep layers of the lamina propria), and *body* (the vocalis muscle).

The *supraglottic vocal tract* includes the pharynx, tongue, palate, oral cavity, nose, and other structures. Together, they act as a *resonator* and are largely responsible for vocal quality or timbre and the perceived character of all speech sounds. The vocal folds themselves produce only a "buzzing" sound.[3] During the course of vocal training for singing, acting, or healthy speaking, changes occur not only in the larynx, but also in the muscle motion, control, and shape of the supraglottic vocal tract.[2]

The *infraglottic vocal tract* (all anatomical structures below the glottis) serves as the *power source* for the voice. Singers and actors refer to the entire power source complex as their "support" or "diaphragm." The anatomy of support for phonation is especially complicated and not completely understood. Yet, it is quite important because deficiencies in support frequently are responsible for voice dysfunction.

The purpose of the support mechanism is to generate a force that directs a controlled airstream between the vocal folds. Active respiratory muscles work in concert with passive forces. The principal muscles of inspiration are the diaphragm (a dome-shaped muscle that extends along the bottom of the rib cage) and the external intercostal muscles (located between the ribs). During quiet respiration, expiration is largely passive. The lungs and rib cage generate passive expiratory forces under many common circumstances such as after a full breath.

Many of the muscles used for active expiration are also employed in "support" for phonation. Muscles of active expiration either raise the intra-abdominal pressure, forcing the diaphragm upward, or lower the ribs or sternum to decrease the dimensions of the thorax, or both, thereby compressing air in the chest. The primary muscles of expiration are "the abdominal muscles," but internal intercostals, and other chest and back muscles are also involved. Trauma or surgery that alters the structure or function of these muscles or ribs undermines the power source of the voice as do diseases, such as asthma, that impair expiration. Deficiencies in the support mechanism often result in compensatory efforts that utilize the laryngeal muscles which are not designed for power source functions. Such behavior can result in decreased function, rapid fatigue, pain, and even structural pathology such as vocal fold nodules.[3] Current expert treatment for such vocal problems focuses on correction of the underlying malfunction rather than surgery.

PHYSIOLOGY OF THE VOICE

The physiology of voice production is extremely complex. Volitional production of voice begins in the cerebral cortex (Fig 2-5). The command

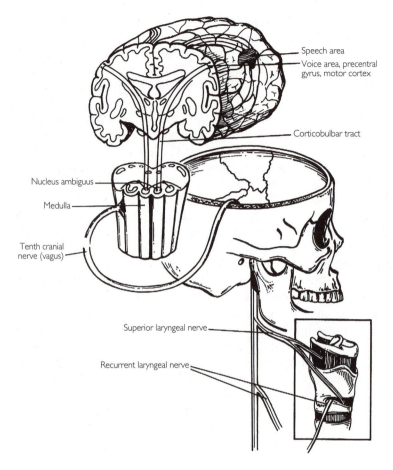

FIGURE 2-5. Simplified summary of pathway for volitional phonation.

for vocalization involves complex interaction among brain centers for speech and other areas. For singing, speech directives must be integrated with information from the centers for musical and artistic expression. The "idea" of the planned vocalization is conveyed to the precentral gyrus in the motor cortex which transmits another set of instructions to the motor nuclei in the brain stem and spinal cord. These areas send out the complicated messages necessary for coordinated activity of the larynx, thoracic and abdominal musculature, and vocal tract articulators. Additional refinement of motor activity is provided by the extrapyramidal and autonomic nervous systems. These impulses combine to produce a sound that is transmitted not only to the ears of the listener, but also to those of the speaker or singer.

Auditory feedback is transmitted from the ear through the brain stem to the cerebral cortex, and adjustments are made which permit the vocalist to match the sound produced with the sound intended, integrating the acoustic properties of the performance environment. Tactile feedback from the throat and muscles involved in phonation is also believed to help in the fine tuning of vocal output, although the mechanism and role of tactile feedback are not fully understood. Many trained singers and speakers cultivate the ability to use tactile feedback effectively because of expected interference with auditory feedback data from ancillary sound such as an orchestra or band.

Phonation, the production of sound, requires interaction among the power source, oscillator, and resonator. The voice may be compared to a brass instrument such as a trumpet. Power is generated by the chest, abdomen, and back musculature and a high-pressure air stream is produced. The trumpeter's lips open and close against the mouthpiece producing a "buzz" similar to the sound produced by vocal fold contact. This sound then passes through the trumpet which has acoustic resonance characteristics that shape the sound we associate with trumpet music. The non-mouthpiece portions of a brass instrument are analogous to the supraglottic vocal tract.

During phonation, the infraglottic musculature must make rapid, complex adjustments because the resistance changes almost continuously as the glottis closes, opens, and changes shape. At the beginning of each phonatory cycle, the vocal folds are approximated, and the glottis is obliterated. This permits infraglottic air pressure to build up, typically to a level of about 7 cm of water, for conversational speech. At this point, the vocal folds are convergent (Fig 2-6A). Because the vocal folds are closed, there is no airflow. The subglottic pressure then pushes the vocal folds progressively farther apart from the bottom up (Fig 2-6B) until a space develops (Fig 2-6C, D) and air begins to flow. Bernoulli force created by the air passes between the vocal folds and combines with the mechanical properties of the folds to begin closing the lower portion of the glottis almost immediately (Fig 2-6E, F, G, H) even while the upper edges are still separating. The principles and mathematics of Bernoulli force are complex. It is a flow effect more easily understood by familiar examples such as the sensation of pull exerted on a vehicle when passed by a truck at high speed or the inward motion of a shower curtain when the water flows past it.

The upper portion of the vocal folds has strong elastic properties which tend to make the vocal folds snap back to the midline. This force becomes more dominant as the upper edges are stretched and the opposing force of the air stream diminishes because of approximation of the lower edges of the vocal folds. The upper portions of the vocal

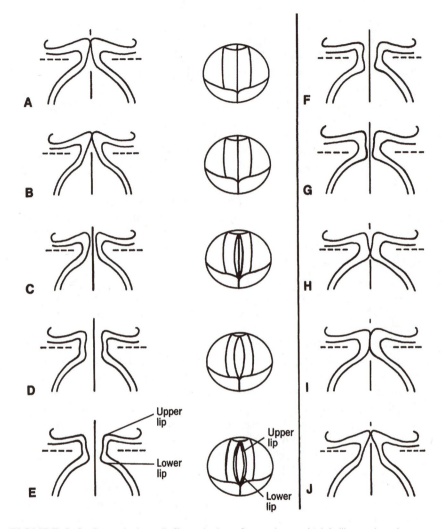

FIGURE 2-6. Frontal view (*left*) and view from above (*right*) illustrating the normal pattern of vocal fold vibration. The vocal fold closes and opens from the inferior aspect of the vibratory margin upwards.

folds are then returned to the midline (Fig 2-6I) completing the glottic cycle. Subglottal pressure then builds again (Fig 2-6J), and the events repeat. The frequency of vibration (number of cycles of openings and closings per second, measured in Hertz [Hz]) is dependent on the air pressure and mechanical properties of the vocal folds which are regulated in part by the laryngeal muscles.[3]

Pitch is the perceptual correlate of frequency. Under most circumstances, as the vocal folds are thinned and stretched and air pressure is increased, the frequency of air pulse emission increases, and pitch goes up. The myoelastic-aerodynamic mechanism of phonation reveals that the vocal folds emit pulses of air, rather than vibrating like strings, and also that there is a vertical phase difference. That is, the lower portion of the vocal folds begins to open and close before the upper portion. The rippling displacement of the vocal fold cover produces a mucosal wave that can be examined clinically under stroboscopic light. If this complex motion is impaired, hoarseness or other changes in voice quality may cause the patient to seek medical evaluation.

The sound produced by the vibrating vocal folds, called the voice source signal, is a complex tone containing a fundamental frequency and many overtones, or higher harmonic partials. The amplitude of the partials decreases uniformly at approximately 12 dB per octave. Interestingly, the acoustic spectrum of the voice source is about the same in ordinary speakers as it is in trained singers and speakers.[2] Voice quality differences in voice professionals occur as the voice source signal passes through their supraglottic vocal tract resonator system (Fig 2-7).

The pharynx, oral cavity, and nasal cavity act as a series of interconnected resonators, which are more complex than that in our trumpet example or other single resonators. As with other resonators, some frequencies are attenuated, others are enhanced. Enhanced frequencies are then radiated with higher relative amplitudes or intensities. Sundberg[1] has shown that the vocal tract has four or five important resonance frequencies called *formants*. The presence of formants alters the uniformly sloping voice source spectrum and creates peaks at formant frequencies. These alterations of the voice source spectral envelope are responsible for distinguishable sounds of speech and song.[2] Formant frequencies are determined by vocal tract shape, which can be altered by the laryngeal, pharyngeal, and oral cavity musculature. Overall vocal tract length and shape are individually fixed and determined by age and sex (females and children have shorter vocal tracts and formant frequencies that are higher than males). Voice training includes conscious physical mastery of the adjustment of vocal tract shape.

Although the formants differ for different vowels, one resonant frequency has received particular attention and is known as the "singer's formant." This formant occurs in the vicinity of 2300 Hz to 3200 Hz for all vowel spectra and appears to be responsible for the "ring" in a singer's or trained speaker's voice. The ability to hear a trained voice clearly even over a loud choir or orchestra is dependent

Generation of Vocal Sound

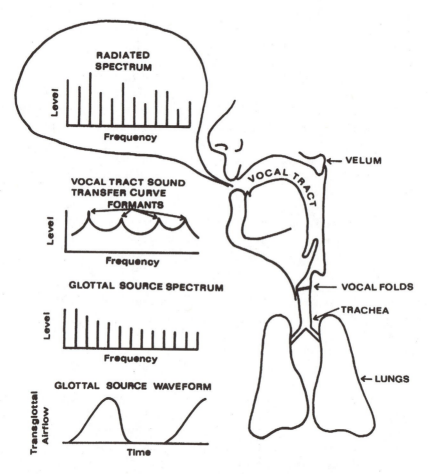

FIGURE 2-7. Determinants of the spectrum of a vowel (oral-output signal).

primarily on the presence of the singer's formant.[1] Interestingly, there is little or no significant difference in maximum vocal intensity between trained and untrained singers. The singer's formant also contributes significantly to the differences in fach (voice classification) among voice categories, occurring in basses at about 2400 Hz, baritones at 2600 Hz, tenors at 2800 Hz, mezzo-sopranos at 2900 Hz, and sopranos at 3200 Hz. It is frequently much less prominent in high soprano singing.[3]

The mechanisms that control two vocal characteristics are particularly important: fundamental frequency and intensity. Fundamental frequency, which corresponds to pitch, can be altered by changing either the air pressure or the mechanical properties of the vocal folds, although the latter is more efficient under most conditions. When the cricothyroid muscle contracts, it makes the thyroid cartilage pivot and increases the distance between the thyroid and arytenoid cartilages, thus stretching the vocal folds. This increases the surface area exposed to subglottal pressure and makes the air pressure more effective in opening the glottis. In addition, stretching of elastic fibers of the vocal fold makes them more efficient at snapping back together. As the cycles shorten and repeat more frequently, the fundamental frequency and pitch rise. Other muscles, including the thyroarytenoid, also contribute.[3] Raising the pressure of the air stream also tends to increase fundamental frequency, a phenomenon for which singers must learn to compensate. Otherwise, their pitch would go up whenever they tried to sing more loudly.

Vocal intensity corresponds to loudness and depends on the degree to which the glottal wave motion excites the air molecules in the vocal tract. Raising the air pressure creates greater amplitude of vocal fold vibration and therefore increases vocal intensity. However, it is actually not the vibration of the vocal fold, but rather the sudden cessation of airflow, that is responsible for initiating acoustic vibration in the vocal tract and controlling intensity. This is similar to the mechanism of acoustic vibration which results from hand clapping. In the larynx, the sharper the cutoff of air flow, the more intense the sound.[3] In the evaluation of voice disorders, an individual's ability to optimize adjustments of air pressure and glottal resistance are assessed. When high subglottic pressure is combined with high adductory (closing) vocal fold force, glottal airflow and the amplitude of the voice source fundamental frequency are low. This is called *pressed phonation* and can be measured clinically through a technique known as flow glottography.[3] Flow glottogram wave amplitude indicates the type of phonation being used, and the slope (closing rate) gives us information about the sound pressure level or loudness. If adductory forces are so weak that the vocal folds do not make contact, the glottis becomes inefficient at resisting air leakage, and the voice source fundamental frequency is also low. This is known as *breathy phonation*. *Flow phonation* is characterized by lower subglottic pressure and lower adductory force. These conditions increase the dominance of the fundamental frequency of the voice source in perceptible sound.[3] Sundberg has shown that the amplitude of the fundamental frequency can be increased by 15 dB or more when the subject changes from pressed phonation to flow phonation.[1] If a patient habitually uses pressed phonation, considerable effort will be required to achieve loud voicing. The muscle patterns and force that are used to compensate for this laryngeal inefficiency may cause vocal damage.

The psychological professional providing care to this population needs a precise (and perhaps new) vocabulary with which to communicate. Many voice patients, especially singers and actors, have fairly good knowledge of voice structure and function. Consequently, the effectiveness and credibility of the clinician are impaired substantially when the psychotherapist does not possess at least a basic understanding of the voice. Rapport is essential to therapeutic communication, regardless of the patient's psychological status. Being able to join, pace, and therefore communicate more effectively within the contextual world of the patient enhances treatment efficacy.

REFERENCES

1. Sundberg J. *The Science of the Singing Voice.* DeKalb, Ill: Northern Illinois University Press; 1987.
2. Scherer RS. Physiology of phonation: a review of basic mechanics. In: Ford CN, Bless DM. *Phonosurgery.* New York, NY: Raven Press; 1991:77-93.
3. Sataloff RT. Clinical anatomy and physiology of the voice. In: Sataloff RT. *Professional Voice: The Science and Art of Clinical Care,* 2nd ed. San Diego, Calif: Singular Publishing Group Inc; 1997.
4. Garrett JD, Larson CR. Neurology of the laryngeal cisson. In: Ford CN, Bless DM. *Phonosurgery.* New York, NY: Raven Press; 1991:43-76.
5. Hirano M. Phonosurgery: basic and clinical investigations. *Otologia* (Fukuoka). 1975;21:239-442.

CHAPTER

3

The Medical History and Physical Examination of the Disordered Voice

In the last 20 years, scientific and technologic advances have resulted in dramatic improvements in medical care of voice disorders. As recently as the 1970s and 1980s, many physicians regarded hoarseness as a symptom of either cancer or "not serious." When benign vocal fold lesions were identified, they usually were treated surgically. This approach often resulted in poor voice quality and recurrent vocal fold masses. Patients without laryngeal masses were likely to be either treated for allergies or told they had "nothing wrong."

In the last several years, attention to a more extensive history, physical examination augmented by new equipment, and better understanding of laryngeal function have increased physicians' awareness of subtle problems in the head and neck that adversely affect the voice, as well as laryngeal manifestations of distant or systemic diseases. Although many of these advances resulted from research inspired by the problems of professional singers and actors, new knowledge has changed the standard of care for all patients with voice complaints.[1,2]

Even minor problems may be particularly apparent in professional singers and actors because of the extreme demands they place on their voices. However, many other patients should be considered voice professionals. They include attorneys, teachers, broadcasters, clergy, sales people, politicians, physicians, shop foremen (who speak over noise), football quarterbacks, secretaries, telephone receptionists, and anyone else whose ability to earn a living is impaired by the presence of voice dysfunction. Because good vocal quality is so significant in professional and personal presentation, all patients should be treated as thoroughly and sensitively as voice professionals.

As discussed in the preceding chapter, the anatomy of the vocal tract is not limited to the larynx. The vocal folds serve as the oscillator of the vocal tract, producing a buzz much like the sound made by a trumpet mouthpiece alone. A delicate balance between intrinsic and extrinsic laryngeal muscle function is important in producing this sound. However, the power source and resonator systems are equally important. The power source consists of the lungs, thorax, and abdominal and back muscles. These structures combine to produce a controlled airstream that passes between the vocal folds. If the power source does not function well, patients tend to compensate for the resulting weakness by hyperfunction of neck muscles not designed for power source functions. This commonly results in voice pathology, such as nodules.[2] Optimal breath support depends on good physical conditioning (particularly respiratory and abdominal muscle function), posture, and other factors.

Once the vocal folds have created the sound by interrupting the airstream passing between them, its quality is shaped by the resonance characteristics of the supraglottic vocal tract. The pharynx, oral cavity, tongue, palate, nose, and, possibly, sinuses are responsible for the harmonic structure of the sound that emanates from the mouth, or its timbre. Consequently, the medical history in any voice patient must take into account not merely the head and neck, but rather the entire body, assessing everything that might cause or aggravate a voice problem.

Extensive review of the medical history for voice patients is beyond the scope of this chapter and is available elsewhere in the literature.[1,2] Psychological professionals are encouraged to consult more extensive discussions of this subject. However, the specific nature of the vocal complaint can be particularly revealing, and all health care providers should seek to establish and understand the reason for voice problems prior to embarking on treatment. Voice patients use the term "hoarseness" to describe a variety of conditions that the physician must separate. Hoarseness is a coarse, scratchy sound most often associated with abnormalities of the vibratory margins of the vocal folds, such as laryngitis, vocal fold hemorrhage, mucosal disruption, mass lesions, and carcinoma.[2]

Breathiness is characterized by excessive loss of air during vocalization. It is often (but not always) associated with hoarseness. In some cases, it is due to improper speaking and/or singing technique. However, any condition that prevents full closure of the vocal folds can be responsible. Such causes include vocal fold paralysis, a mass separating the leading edges of the vocal folds, arthritis of the cricoarytenoid joints, arytenoid dislocation, and senile vocal fold atrophy. Forced breathiness (a strained whisper) is often, but not always, a manifestation of psychogenic dysphonia or malingering.

Fatigue of the voice is inability to continue speaking or singing for extended periods without a change in voice quality. The voice may fatigue by becoming hoarse, changing in timbre, "cracking," breaking into different registers, or manifesting other uncontrolled aberrations. Fatigue often is caused by misuse of abdominal and neck musculature. Vocal fatigue also may be a sign of generalized malaise or serious illness, such as myasthenia gravis or chronic fatigue syndrome.[2]

Volume disturbance may present as inability to speak or sing loudly, or softly. Each voice has its own inherent dynamic range, although this can be improved through voice training. Most volume problems in patients who are not professional voice users are due to technical errors. However, hormonal changes, aging, and neurologic disease also may alter voice volume. Paralysis of the superior laryngeal nerve will impair the ability to speak loudly and project the voice. Damage to this nerve is a frequently unrecognized consequence of herpes and other viral infections.

Prolonged vocal warm-up time is most often associated with gastroesophageal reflux laryngitis, a condition in which the sphincter between the stomach and esophagus is inefficient, and stomach secretions reach up into the larynx. "Tickling" or choking during singing suggests a problem on the vibratory margin of the vocal folds, particularly laryngitis or voice abuse. In this case, the vocal folds should be visualized by the physician before additional phonation is attempted. Pain while speaking or singing can indicate vocal fold lesions, laryngeal joint arthritis, infection, or reflux; but it is much more commonly caused by voice abuse with excessive muscle activity in the neck. This symptom does not usually require immediate cessation of phonation pending medical examination.[2]

After determining the time of onset and nature of the voice complaint, the patient's age, vocal demands, and the professional importance of the voice, as well as a preliminary survey of the voice problems of the individual, an exhaustive history is necessary. Appendix II contains a summary of the questions routinely asked of professional singers in our voice center. Professional and nonprofessional singers and speakers undergo the same inquiry, except for the addition of questions specifically relevant to singing or acting performance. The history investigates voice training; vocal skills; professional status,

goals, and commitments; the nature and timing of pressing professional voice commitments; the consequences of canceling commitments;
family vocal history (including disorders and particular excellence);
and all aspects of general health.

Patients also are questioned about laryngeal trauma including external injuries and internal injuries caused by voice abuse or misuse.
Medical health questions investigate problems related to various medical conditions including infections (such as laryngitis, tonsillitis, sinusitis, head colds); allergies; substance abuse (including smoking); respiratory dysfunction; hormonal problems (such as premenstrual vocal
difficulties, or hypothyroidism); gastroenterologic problems such as reflux; skeletal problems that may alter posture and support or cause tension (such as limb, back or neck problems including whiplash); dental
dysfunction that may cause temporomandibular joint pain which alters
the voice by adding muscular tension to the vocal mechanism; neurological problems; and injury.[2] The details of this process are apparent
from the questionnaires, and the reasons for such an inquiry will become clearer in the following chapter on common diagnoses and treatments of vocal dysfunction.

Familiarity with the inquiry process and the information it reveals is
extremely valuable to the medical psychologist; and all psychological
professionals who become active in caring for voice patients, especially
singers and actors, are strongly advised to learn more about medical
care of voice disorders. The body and mind are intimately linked in all
health and disease. Responsible collaboration as a member of a voice
team requires familiarity with the medical and behavioral treatment
provided to the patient by colleagues. This is best acquired by extensive
study and spending time in a medical center becoming personally familiar with medical history taking, examination, and treatment approaches.

PHYSICAL EXAMINATION

Every patient with a voice complaint should have a complete otolaryngologic examination, vocal fold visualization, at least by indirect mirror
laryngoscopy, and more general medical examination as indicated. Examination of the ears should include assessment of hearing acuity, as
even a relatively slight hearing loss may lead a patient to speak or sing
at increased volume, resulting in voice strain. This problem is prominent primarily in sensorineural hearing loss. The conjunctivae of the
eyes should be observed for signs of allergy, anemia, jaundice, and other abnormalities that may underlie the voice complaint.

The nose should be assessed for patency of the nasal airway. Nasal breathing is optimal because it allows filtration, warming, and humidification of air before it reaches the vocal folds. Nasal obstruction necessitates mouth breathing, which may increase mucosal irritation and drying.

Oral cavity examination should include special note of xerostomia (excessively dry mucous membranes), dental wear patterns, and transparency of the enamel of the central incisors of the teeth. Thinning of incisor enamel may be caused by frequent contact with gastric acid in patients with bulimia. The history of bulimia is rarely volunteered, and physical signs offer the physician an opportunity to question the patient more carefully about this potential diagnosis. The condition often produces laryngeal symptoms and signs indistinguishable from gastroesophageal reflux laryngitis.

Neck examination should include special attention to the thyroid gland and to the posterior portion of the neck for excessive muscle tension or limitation of range of motion. Neck pain and muscular hyperfunction often are associated with voice fatigue and altered function. Cranial nerve examination should also be included with particular attention to gag reflex (especially with a history of herpetic cold sores), deviation of the palate, or other mild cranial nerve deficits that may indicate injury to cranial nerves. Neuropathies resulting from postviral infection often involve the superior laryngeal nerve and cause voice weakness, loss of projection, instability, and trouble maintaining higher pitches.[3]

Laryngeal examination begins when the patient enters the physician's office. The range, ease, volume, and quality of the speaking voice should be noted during conversational speech. If the patient is a singer or actor, the voice should also be evaluated during simulated performance. Specific techniques for assessing the voice during speaking or singing are described elsewhere.[2,3]

The current standard of medical care requires that indirect laryngoscopy be performed on every patient with a voice complaint. This technique, which has been used since 1854, allows the larynx to be visualized with a small long-handled mirror and a reflected light source. It is still excellent for assessing symmetry of vocal fold abduction and adduction, laryngeal color, and the presence of substantial masses or lesions. However, it does not provide an adequate physical examination of the vibratory margin.[3]

When phonating at the pitch middle C, the vocal folds are vibrating at 250 times per second. The eye cannot detect many important lesions that impair vibration and produce hoarseness and breathiness without slow motion evaluation. This evaluation is now possible routinely through strobovideolaryngoscopy.

The stroboscopic light is usually triggered using a laryngeal microphone. Flexible nasal fiberoptic laryngoscopes and magnifying rigid laryngeal telescopes are used during a series of vocal tasks to permit evaluation of the vibratory margin. This technique allows diagnosis of vocal fold scarring, small masses, neurologic abnormalities, and early cancers that are missed by indirect laryngoscopy with continuous light.[4,5] Stroboscopy is now available in an increasing number of otolaryngology centers throughout the United States and elsewhere.

Reliable, valid, objective analysis of the voice is also extremely important. The equivalent of the audiometer used to assess hearing does not exist for voice yet, but many procedures and instruments for voice quantification are available. They are extremely helpful for diagnostic purposes and for assessment of the results of medical, behavioral, and surgical treatment. Assessment of vibration is accomplished through strobovideolaryngoscopy, electroglottography, photoglottography, and other techniques. Electroglottography creates a wave that represents vocal fold contact (the closing glottis) by passing a small electrical current through two surface electrodes in contact with the skin of the neck. Photoglottography documents the opening glottis using a light passed between the vocal folds.[2]

Measures of phonatory ability are the easiest and most readily available. Maximum phonation time can be measured using a stopwatch, instructing the patient to sustain the vowel /ɑ/ at a comfortable frequency and intensity (which should be measured and noted) for as long as possible following a deep inspiration. Frequency and intensity ranges also can be measured easily.[2]

Acoustic analysis requires more extensive equipment but gives information about spectral harmonics, amount of noise in the sound signal, cycle-to-cycle perturbations, and other useful characteristics. Aerodynamic measures are especially important and can be performed with routine pulmonary function equipment. They include traditional pulmonary function testing and measures of laryngeal airflow performed using a spirometer and specific phonatory tasks. Laryngeal electromyography (direct measurement of nerve function) and formal psychoacoustic evaluation complete the current battery of comprehensive voice evaluation.[2]

Through comprehensive history, physical examination, and testing, it is now generally possible to establish accurately the organic basis for voice complaints. In a subspecialty practice, this process routinely involves evaluation by a laryngologist, speech-language pathologist, and usually a singing voice specialist (singing teacher trained to work with injured voices). In most cases, it also includes evaluation by an acting voice trainer and at least cursory assessment by a psychological professional. The entire voice team is sensitive to the psychological problems that may cause or arise in association with voice disorders. The potential need for formal assessment and treatment by a psychological professional is considered in every patient with voice complaints. It is not unusual to identify significant psychopathology; and it is common to discover marked anxiety and stress that benefit from formal intervention.

REFERENCES

1. Sataloff RT. The professional voice: Part I: Anatomy and history. *J Voice.* 1987;1(1):92-104.
2. Sataloff RT. *Professional Voice: The Science and Art of Clinical Care,* 2nd ed. San Diego, Calif: Singular Publishing Group Inc; 1997.
3. Sataloff RT. The professional voice: Part II: Physical examination. *J Voice.* 1987;1(2):191-201.
4. Sataloff RT, Spiegel JR, Carroll LM, et al. Strobovideolaryngoscopy in professional voice users: results, findings and clinical value. *J Voice.* 1988;1(4):359-364.
5. Sataloff RT, Spiegel JR, Hawkshaw MJ. Strobovideolaryngoscopy: results and clinical value. *Ann Otol Rhinol Laryngol.* 1991;100(9):725-727.

CHAPTER

4

Common Diagnoses and Interdisciplinary Treatment in Professional Voice Users

Numerous medical conditions adversely affect the voice. Many have their origins primarily outside the head and neck. This chapter is not intended to be all inclusive, but rather to introduce some of the more common and important conditions found in professional voice users seeking medical care.

VOICE ABUSE

Speaking in noisy environments, such as cars and airplanes, is particularly abusive to the voice. So are backstage greetings, postperformance parties, choral conducting, voice teaching, and cheerleading. With proper training, all of these activities can be done safely. However, most patients, surprisingly even singers, have little or no training for the speaking voice.

If voice abuse is caused by speech, treatment should be provided by a licensed, certified speech-language pathologist. In many cases, training the speaking voice will benefit singers greatly not only by improving speech, but also by helping singing technique. Physicians should not hesitate to recommend such training, but it should be performed by an expert speech-language pathologist who specializes in voice. Many speech-language pathologists who are well trained in swallowing rehabilitation, articulation therapy, and other techniques are not expert in voice therapy.

Specialized singing training also may be helpful to some voice patients who are not singers. Initial singing training teaches relaxation techniques, develops muscle strength, and is symbiotic with standard speech therapy.

Abuse of the voice during singing is a complex problem. When voice abuse is suspected or observed in a patient with vocal complaints, he or she should be referred to a laryngologist who specializes in voice, preferably a physician affiliated with a voice care team.

STRUCTURAL ABNORMALITIES

Vocal Nodules

Nodules are callouslike masses of the vocal folds which are caused by vocally abusive behaviors. Occasionally, laryngoscopic evaluation reveals asymptomatic vocal nodules that do not appear to interfere with voice production. Some famous and successful singers have had untreated vocal nodules. If the nodules are asymptomatic, they should not be disturbed. However, in most cases, nodules result in hoarseness, breathiness, loss of range, and vocal fatigue. They may be due to abuse of the speaking voice, the singing voice, or both.

Voice therapy should always be utilized as the initial therapeutic modality and will cure the majority of patients. Even apparently large, fibrotic nodules often shrink, disappear, or become asymptomatic with 6 to 12 weeks of voice therapy if the patient complies with instructions. Even in patients who eventually need surgical excision of their nodules, preoperative voice therapy is essential to prevent recurrence.[1]

The use of the laser remains controversial among laryngologists who perform vocal fold surgery. Some evidence indicates that laser therapy results in a longer healing time and a higher incidence of vocal fold scar and poor voice.[2,3] Other laryngologists believe that, if high wattage and short duration bursts are used, these surgical complications should not occur any more often than with conventional surgical treatment.[2,3]

In any case, it is essential that excision of vocal fold masses be superficial. These lesions are not malignant (although tissue should be obtained for histologic study by a pathologist regardless of whether a laser is used), and there is no need to cut a divot out of the vocal fold. If the lesions are removed to a level even with the vocal fold edge and the underlying lamina propria is disturbed as little as possible, scarring will be minimized. This principle holds for use of laser as well as traditional instrumentation.

Vocal Polyps

Vocal polyps, another type of benign vocal fold mass, are usually single lesions. Often, examination with a microscope will reveal a feeding vessel on the vocal fold, usually on the upper surface. Polyps may disappear spontaneously, but they often require surgical excision. A trial of speech therapy, low-dose steroids, and reexamination in 4 weeks produces surprising resolution in some patients. When surgery is necessary, the lesion is excised with minimal disruption of the mucosa along the leading edge of the vocal fold, and cauterization of the feeding vessel with 1-watt laser bursts may help prevent recurrence. This technique is also useful in the treatment of recurrent vocal fold hemorrhages. In all laryngeal surgery, delicate microscopic dissection is now the standard of care. Vocal fold "stripping," an out-of-date surgical approach formerly used for benign lesions, often resulted in scar and poor voice function. It is no longer an acceptable technique.[4,5]

Vocal Fold Cysts

Submucosal lesions of the vocal fold, such as cysts, usually do not resolve spontaneously. They may be excised using a small, superficial incision along the superior edge. Superficial submucosal dissection allows removal of the cyst without disruption of the leading edge. Care should be taken not to disturb normal tissues adjacent to the lesion.[1]

Reinke's Edema

Reinke's edema is characterized by an "elephant ear," floppy vocal fold appearance. It is also observed during examination in many nonprofessional voice users and is accompanied by a low, coarse, gruff voice. It is seen less frequently among pop singers, radio and sports broadcasters, attorneys, and other professional voice users and rarely in classical singers. Reinke's edema is nearly always associated with cigarette smoking, although other factors, such as hypothyroidism and voice abuse, may be present. If it does not resolve after all irritants have been removed and voice technique has been modified, surgery may be necessary.

When vocal fold surgery is performed, only one vocal fold should be operated on at a time. The vocal fold may be incised along its superior surface and the edematous material removed with a fine suction. This procedure often produces a very satisfactory voice, and it may be unnecessary to operate on the opposite vocal fold even at a later date. Career concerns must be a component of the caution exercised in treating this condition, particularly in professional voice users; and patients must fully understand the benefits and risks of treatment. In an actor or radio announcer, for example, the edema may be partially responsible for the performer's "vocal signature." Restoring the voice to a satisfactory cosmetic appearance and "normal" sound may damage or end a performer's career.

Cancer

A detailed discussion of cancer of the vocal folds is beyond the scope of this chapter. The prognosis for small vocal fold cancers is good, whether they are treated by radiation or surgery. Although it may seem intuitively obvious that radiation therapy provides a better chance of voice conservation than even limited vocal fold surgery, later radiation changes in the vocal fold may produce substantial hoarseness, xerophonia (dry voice), and voice dysfunction. Consequently, from the standpoint of voice preservation, optimal treatments remain uncertain.[5 (pp307-310)]

Prospective studies using objective voice measures and strobovideolaryngoscopy should answer the relevant questions in the near future. Strobovideolaryngoscopy is also valuable for follow-up of patients who have had laryngeal cancers. It permits detection of microscopic vibratory changes associated with infiltration by the cancer long before they can be seen with continuous light. Stroboscopy has been used in Europe and Japan for this purpose for many years. In the United States, the popularity of strobovideolaryngoscopy for follow-up of cancer patients has increased greatly in the last 5 years.[5 (pp307-310)]

The psychological consequences of vocal fold cancer can be devastating, especially in a professional voice user. They may be overwhelming for nonvoice professionals, as well. These reactions are understandable and expected. In many patients, however, psychological reactions may be as severe following medically "less significant" vocal fold problems such as hemorrhages, nodules, and other conditions that do not command the public respect and sympathy afforded to a cancer. In many ways, the management of related psychological problems can be even more difficult in patients with these "lesser" vocal disturbances.

INFECTION AND INFLAMMATION

Tonsillitis

Recurrent tonsillitis in professional voice users is particularly problematic. On the one hand, surgeons are not anxious to perform a tonsillectomy on an established voice professional because of the potential for effects on vocal quality associated with supraglottic resonance changes. On the other hand, a professional who depends on his or her voice cannot afford to be sick for a week five or six times a year. Such incapacitation is damaging to income and reputation.

In general, the same conservative approach toward treatment of recurrent tonsillitis used in other patients should be applied to professional voice users, but tonsillectomy should not be withheld if it is really indicated. During surgery, it is particularly important to remove only the tonsil itself without damaging the surrounding tissues to minimize restriction of palatal and pharyngeal motion by scar formation. The patient must be warned that tonsillectomy may alter the sound of his or her voice. This is not usually a major problem, but it can be.

In addition to recurrent, acute tonsillitis, halitosis (foul breath) caused by accumulated debris in tonsillar crypts may be an appropriate indication for tonsillectomy. Gastroesophageal reflux, dental disease, metabolic abnormalities, and other causes of halitosis must be ruled out. If chronic tonsillitis has been established as the etiology, surgical treatment can be offered. Although halitosis is not ordinarily considered a serious malady, it may be a major impediment to success for people who have to work in close physical proximity to others, such as singers, actors, dentists, barbers, some physicians, psychologists, and so on. If the problem cannot be cured with medication or with oral cavity hygiene using a soft toothbrush or water spray to cleanse the tonsil, tonsillectomy may be reasonable.

Upper Respiratory Tract Infection Without Laryngitis

Although mucosal irritation usually is diffuse in upper tracheal infections, patients sometimes describe marked nasal obstruction with little or no sore throat and a "normal" voice. If the laryngeal examination shows no abnormality, the patient with a "head cold" may be permitted to speak or sing. However, the patient should be advised by the laryngologist not to try to duplicate his or her usual sound, but rather to accept the insurmountable alterations caused by changes in the supraglottic vocal tract. The patient is cautioned against throat clearing, because it is traumatic to the tissues and may produce laryngitis. If a cough is present, nonnarcotic medications may be prescribed to suppress it. The decision as to whether it is advisable for the professional voice user to perform under these circumstances then rests with the performer and his or her business associates. Performers may manifest stress responses and require cognitive support to make assertive, prudent decisions.

Laryngitis With Serious Vocal Fold Injury

Hemorrhage in the vocal fold and mucosal disruption are *contraindications* to speaking or singing. When these findings are observed, medical treatment includes strict voice rest in addition to correction of any underlying disease. Vocal fold hemorrhage in skilled voice users is seen most commonly in premenstrual women using aspirin products. Severe hemorrhage with consequent mucosal scarring may result in permanent alterations in vocal fold vibratory function. In rare instances, surgical intervention may be necessary.

The potential gravity of these conditions must be stressed, because many people, especially performers including politicians and clergy, are reluctant to stop speaking or singing. At the present time, acute treatment of vocal fold hemorrhage is medically controversial. Most laryngologists allow the hematoma (blood clot) to resolve spontaneously. Because this sometimes results in an organized hematoma and scar formation requiring later surgery; in selected cases, some physicians advocate making an incision along the superior edge of the vocal fold and draining the hematoma. Further study is ongoing to determine the optimal therapeutic approach.

Laryngitis Without Serious Vocal Fold Damage

Mild to moderate edema and erythema of the vocal folds may result from infection or noninfectious causes. When there is no evidence of mucosal disruption or hemorrhage, these findings are not absolute prohibitions to voice use. Noninfectious laryngitis commonly occurs in association with excessive voice use. It may also be caused by other forms of vocally abusive behavior and by mucosal irritation due to allergy, smoke inhalation, and other causes.

Thick, tenacious strands of mucus visible on examination between the anterior and middle thirds of the vocal folds are often indicative of voice abuse. "Laryngitis sicca" is associated with dehydration, dry atmosphere, mouth breathing, and antihistamine therapy. Deficiency of lubrication causes irritation and coughing and results in mild inflammation.

If there is no pressing professional need for performance, inflammatory conditions of the larynx are usually treated by the laryngologist with relative voice rest in addition to other medical modalities. However, in some instances, voice use is permitted. These patients are then instructed to avoid all forms of irritation and to rest their voices at all times except when speaking or singing is urgent professionally. Corticosteroids and other medications discussed later in this book may be helpful. If mucosal secretions are excessive, low-dose antihistamine therapy may be beneficial, but it is prescribed with caution and generally avoided. Copious, thin secretions are better for the voice than scant, thick secretions or excessive dryness. The vocalist with laryngitis must stay very well hydrated to maintain the desired character of mucosal lubrication.

Infectious laryngitis may be caused by bacteria or viruses. Involvement of the tissues below the larynx frequently is indicative of a more severe infection which may be difficult to control medically in a short period of time. Indiscriminate use of antibiotics is avoided by physicians, but patients will often "self-medicate," choosing ineffective drugs or dosage regimens. When the physician is in doubt as to the cause and a major voice commitment is imminent, vigorous antibiotic treatment is warranted. In this circumstance, the damage caused by allowing progression of a curable condition is greater than the damage that might result from a course of therapy for an unproven microorganism while culture results are pending.

Voice rest (absolute or relative) is an important therapeutic consideration in any case of laryngitis. When there are no pressing professional commitments, a short course of absolute voice rest may be suggested by the laryngologist because it is the safest and most conservative therapeutic intervention. This means absolute silence and communication with a writing pad. The patient is instructed not even to whisper, because this may be an even more traumatic vocal activity than speaking softly. Whistling through the lips also requires laryngeal activity and should not be permitted. The prescription of absolute voice rest may provoke psychological decompensation in some susceptible individuals. It mirrors claustrophobic isolation and evokes anxiety responses.

Absolute voice rest (silence) is necessary only for serious vocal fold injury, such as hemorrhage or mucosal disruption. Even then, it is virtually never required for more than 7 to 10 days. A 3-day period is often sufficient. Some excellent laryngologists do not believe voice rest is necessary at all. However, absolute voice rest for a few days is thought to be helpful in some patients with laryngitis, especially gregarious, verbal singers and actors who find it difficult to moderate their voice use to comply with instructions for relative voice rest.

In many instances, considerations of economics and reputation militate against a medical recommendation for voice rest. In such cases, patients are instructed to speak softly, as infrequently as possible, and often at a slightly higher pitch than usual; to avoid excessive telephone use; and to speak with abdominal support as they would use in singing. This is the technique of relative voice rest, and it is helpful in most cases.

An urgent session with a speech-language pathologist is also extremely helpful in providing guidelines to prevent voice abuse and often will be arranged during a patient's visit to the laryngologist. Nevertheless, the patient must be made aware by the physician that there is some increased risk associated with performing with laryngitis. Inflammation of the vocal folds produces increased capillary fragility and increased risk of vocal fold injury or hemorrhage. Many factors must be considered by the patient and physician in determining whether a given commitment is important enough to justify the potential consequences to long-term vocal health. Performers experience this as a crisis to their career and reputation. At the same time, they fear damage to their "vocal instrument." Immobilization, impaired cognition, and labile affect may be evident. Crisis intervention strategies by the psychological professional may be required.

Steam inhalations which deliver moisture and heat to the vocal folds and tracheobronchial tree are often useful. Nasal irrigations are used by some people, but have little scientifically proven value. Gargling also has no proven efficacy, but it is probably harmful only if it involves loud, abusive vocalization as part of the gargling process. Ultrasonic moisture treatments, local massage, brief psychotherapy, and biofeedback directed at relieving anxiety and decreasing muscle tension may be helpful adjuncts to a broader treatment program. However, psychotherapy and biofeedback, if prescribed, must be delivered expertly. Voice lessons given by a singing teacher experienced in working with vocal impairment combined with speech therapy are invaluable, once the patient is permitted to phonate.[1]

Sinusitis

Chronic inflammation of the mucosa lining the sinus cavities commonly produces thick secretions known as postnasal drip. Postnasal drip can be particularly problematic because it causes excessive phlegm which interferes with phonation, and because it leads to frequent throat clearing which may inflame the vocal folds.[1] Sometimes chronic sinusitis is caused by allergies and can be treated with medications. However, many medications used for this condition cause side effects that are unacceptable in professional voice users, particularly mucosal drying. When medication management is not satisfactory, functional endoscopic sinus surgery may be appropriate.[1] Acute purulent sinusitis is a different matter. It requires aggressive treatment with antibiotics, sometimes surgical drainage, treatment of underlying conditions (such as dental abscess), and occasionally surgery.[1]

SYSTEMIC CONDITIONS

Aging

Advanced age produces normal changes throughout the voice-producing mechanism. Abdominal and general muscle tone decrease, lungs lose elasticity, the thorax loses distensibility, the mucosa of the vocal tract atrophies, mucous secretions change character, nerve endings are reduced in number, and psychoneurologic functions differ. The larynx itself loses muscle tone and bulk and may show depletion of submucosal ground substance in the vocal fold when examined histologically. The laryngeal cartilages ossify (turn to bone), and the joints become arthritic and stiffen. The hormonal environment changes throughout the body.

The effects of the changes of aging seem to be more pronounced in female vocalists. Males are more likely to extend their vocal careers into their seventies.[6,7] However, some degree of breathiness and other aging changes should be expected in most elderly patients. Estrogen replacement may forestall by many years the appearance of disturbing changes in postmenopausal singers. However, it should not be given alone. Sequential replacement is most physiologic.[8,9]

Respiratory Dysfunction

Respiratory impairment is especially problematic to singers and other voice professionals,[10] and also for wind instrumentalists. Breath support is essential to healthy voice production. The effects of severe *respiratory infection* are well understood and will not be enumerated. *Restrictive lung disease*, such as that associated with obesity, may impair breath support by decreasing lung volume and respiratory efficiency. Even mild *obstructive lung disease* (such as asthma or emphysema) can impair breath support enough to result in increased neck and tongue muscle tension, and abusive voice use capable of producing vocal nodules.[10]

This scenario occurs in patients with unrecognized asthma. The condition may be difficult for the physician to diagnose unless it is suspected, because many such cases of asthma are exercise-induced (voice performance is a form of exercise), and respiratory performance may be normal at rest during medical evaluation. Consequently, the singer or animated speaker has normal pulmonary function clinically and may even have reasonably normal pulmonary function tests at rest in the physician's office. He or she will also usually support the voice well and sing with good technique during the first portion of a performance. However, as performance exercise continues, pulmonary function decreases, effectively impairing support, and resulting in abusive technique.[1,10]

When suspected, this entity can be confirmed through a methacholine challenge test in which pulmonary function testing is performed before and after administration of a drug known to produce airway narrowing in susceptible individuals. Treatment of the underlying pulmonary disease to restore the ability to utilize effective support is essential for resolving the vocal problem. Treating asthma is more difficult in professional voice users because of the need in some patients to avoid not only inhalers, but also drugs that produce even a mild tremor, which may be audible during soft singing or speaking. Consultant management by a skilled pulmonologist who specializes in asthma treatment and who is sensitive to the problems of performing artists is extremely helpful.

Allergy

Mild allergies are more incapacitating to professional voice users than to others because of their effects on the mucosal cover layer of the vocal folds. In patients who have only short periods of annual allergy and are able to control the symptoms satisfactorily with antihistamines that do not produce disturbing side effects, drug therapy is satisfactory. When used, very mild antihistamines in small doses should be tried. The physician and patient must often "experiment" with several antihistamines before finding a suitable balance between therapeutic effect and side effects. The adverse side effects may be counteracted to some extent with mucolytic drugs which thin mucous secretions. However, allergy medications produce sufficient difficulty especially in professional voice users to warrant thorough allergic evaluation and hyposensitization therapy ("allergy shots") in many patients who might not need to undergo this process if they were in professions less dependent on vocal quality and endurance.

Gastroesophageal Reflux Laryngitis

Gastroesophageal reflux laryngitis is extremely common among voice patients. This is a condition in which the sphincter between the stomach and esophagus is inefficient, and acidic stomach secretions reach the laryngeal tissues causing inflammation. The most typical symptoms are hoarseness in the morning, prolonged vocal warm-up time, halitosis and a bitter taste in the morning, a feeling of a "lump in the throat," frequent throat clearing, chronic irritative cough, and frequent tracheitis or tracheobronchitis. Any or all of these symptoms may be present. Heartburn is not common in these patients, so the diagnosis is often missed.

Physical examination usually reveals erythema (redness) of the arytenoid mucosa. A barium swallow radiographic study with water siphonage may provide additional information, but is not needed routinely. However, if a patient complies strictly with treatment recommendations and does not show marked improvement within a month, or if there is a reason to suspect more serious pathology, complete evaluation by a gastroenterologist should be carried out. Twenty-four hour pH monitoring of the esophagus and pharynx is often most effective in establishing a diagnosis. The results are correlated with a diary of the patient's activities and symptoms. Bulimia should also be considered in the differential diagnosis when symptoms are refractory to treatment and other physical and psychological signs are suggestive.[1]

The mainstays of treatment for reflux laryngitis are elevation of the head of the bed (not just sleeping on pillows), antacids, H-2 blockers or proton pump inhibitors, and avoidance of eating for 3 to 4 hours before going to sleep. This is often difficult for singers and actors because of their performance schedule, but if they are counseled about minor changes in eating habits (such as eating larger meals at breakfast and lunch), they usually can comply. Avoidance of alcohol, caffeine, and specific foods is beneficial. Medications that decrease or block acid production may be necessary and are further discussed in Chapter 5.

Hypothyroidism

The human voice is particularly sensitive to endocrinologic changes. Many of these changes involve alterations of fluid content beneath the laryngeal mucosa, which affect the bulk and shape of the vocal folds and result in audible voice change. Hypothyroidism is a well-recognized cause of voice disorders, although the mechanism is not well understood.[11-13] Hoarseness, vocal fatigue, muffling, loss of range, a feeling of a lump in the throat, and a sensation of a "veil over the voice" may be present even with mild hypothyroidism.

Even when thyroid function blood test results are within the low-normal range, this diagnosis will be entertained by the experienced laryngologist, especially if thyroid-stimulating hormone blood levels are in the high-normal range or are elevated. A therapeutic trial of thyroid hormone replacement is often prescribed under these circumstances, especially if the patient is overweight or has other clinical signs of borderline thyroid function. Thyrotoxicosis (extreme elevations in thyroid hormone levels) may result in similar voice disturbances.[14]

Laryngopathia Premenstrualis and Laryngopathia Gravidarum

Voice changes associated with sex hormone levels are encountered often in medical practices which specialize in voice care. Although they may be significant occasionally in men, voice problems related to sex hormones are seen most commonly in females. Most of the ill-effects occur in the immediate premenstrual period and are known as "laryngopathia premenstrualis." This common condition is caused by physiologic, anatomic, and emotional alterations secondary to endocrine changes. The vocal dysfunction described is characterized by decreased vocal efficiency, and some "muffling" of the voice. It is most troublesome in singers and is often more apparent to the singer than to the listener. Submucosal hemorrhages in the larynx are more common during this time.[15]

In many European opera houses, singers used to be excused from singing during the premenstrual and early menstrual days through "grace days" specified in their contracts, but this practice is not followed in the United States and is being abandoned in Europe. Ovulation-inhibiting agents may mitigate some of these symptoms,[16] but in some women, birth control pills deleteriously alter voice range and character after only a few months of use.[17-20] These changes are usually reversible if the medication is discontinued. When oral contraceptives are used, the voice must be monitored closely by the laryngologist and patient. Under crucial performance circumstances, oral contraceptive agents may be prescribed to alter the time of menstruation, but this practice is justified only in the most extraordinary situations.[18-20]

The hormonal environment of pregnancy frequently results in voice alterations known as "laryngopathia gravidarum." The changes may be similar to those noted premenstrually or may be perceived as desirable changes. In some cases, alterations produced by pregnancy are permanent.[21,22]

Although hormonally induced changes in the larynx and respiratory mucosa secondary to menstruation and pregnancy are discussed widely in the medical literature, insufficient attention has been paid by practitioners to the important alterations in abdominal support that may occur. Dysmenorrhea (the muscle cramping associated with menstruation) causes pain and hinders abdominal function. Abdominal distension during pregnancy also changes abdominal musculature. Any professional voice user whose abdominal support is compromised will usually be discouraged by her laryngologist from performing until the abdominal impairment is resolved. People who must speak extensively, such as teachers, should be counseled to be alert for voice fatigue, especially during the last trimester.

Under no circumstances should androgens be given to female voice professionals, even in small amounts, if there is any therapeutic alternative. Androgens are found in common medications used for endometriosis. If prescribed, patients must be warned about potential voice changes, and informed consent should be obtained. Androgens cause unsteadiness of the voice, rapid changes of timbre, and lowering of the fundamental frequency. This masculinization is similar to the changes observed during voice maturation of male children at puberty. The changes are irreversible. Drug preparations with progestins should be used instead of androgen preparations whenever medically possible. In rare instances, endogenous androgens may be produced by pathologic conditions, such as ovarian or adrenal tumors, and voice alterations may be among the first presenting symptoms.[6,7,23-27]

Poor General Health

As with any other athletic activity, optimal voice use requires reasonably good general health and physical conditioning. Abdominal and respiratory strength and endurance are particularly important. If a professional voice user becomes short of breath from climbing two flights of stairs, he or she certainly does not have the physical stamina necessary for proper respiratory support for a speech, let alone a strenuous musical production. This deficiency usually results in abusive vocal habits used in vain attempts to compensate for the deficiencies.

General illnesses, such as anemia, mononucleosis, AIDS, chronic fatigue syndrome, or other diseases associated with malaise and weakness may impair the ability of vocal musculature to recover rapidly from heavy use and may also be associated with alterations of mucosal secretions. Other systemic illnesses may be responsible for voice complaints, particularly if they impair the abdominal muscles necessary for breath support. For example, diarrhea and constipation that prohibit sustained abdominal contraction may be reasons for the physician to prohibit a strenuous singing or acting engagement.

Any extremity injury, such as a sprained ankle, may alter posture and therefore interfere with customary abdominothoracic support. Voice patients are often unaware of this problem and develop abusive, hyperfunctional compensatory maneuvers in the neck and tongue musculature as a result. These technical flaws may produce voice complaints, such as vocal fatigue and neck pain, that bring the performer to the physician's office for assessment and care.

PSYCHOLOGICAL CONSIDERATIONS

Anxiety

Voice patients frequently are sensitive and communicative people. When the principal cause of vocal dysfunction is anxiety, the skilled laryngologist often can deliver initial treatment with a few minutes of assurance that there is no organic difficulty on the larynx and by stating the diagnosis of anxiety reaction. The patient should be counseled that anxiety reactions are common, especially in professional voice users. Recognition of anxiety as the principal problem frequently allows the performer to overcome it using his or her customary coping responses.

Tranquilizers and sedatives are rarely necessary and are undesirable because they may interfere with fine motor control. A review of the medications available for treatment of psychologic disorders is presented in Chapter 5. Although these drugs have a place under occasional, extraordinary circumstances, their routine use is not only potentially hazardous in professional voice users, but also violates an important therapeutic principle. Performers have chosen a career that exposes them to the public. If such a person is so incapacitated by anxiety that he or she is unable to perform the routine functions of his or her chosen profession without chemical help, this should be considered symptomatic of a significant underlying psychologic problem that warrants referral. If such a dependence exists, evaluation by an experienced arts-medicine psychologist or psychiatrist should be provided promptly. Obscuring the symptoms by fostering the dependence is not only insufficient, but dangerous.

Hypochondriasis

Hypochondriasis is fairly uncommon among patients with voice disorders in the general population; and it is extremely rare in professional voice users, especially singers and actors. Performance careers are bound to a "show must go on" ethic. These professions will not tolerate people who chronically complain and repeatedly cancel. In general, failure to establish a medical diagnosis in a professional voice user is more often due to lack of expertise and breadth of therapeutic investigation on the part of the physician than an imaginary complaint.

Other Psychological Problems

Psychogenic voice disorders, incapacitating psychological reactions to organic voice disorders, and other psychological problems are encountered fairly commonly among voice patients. They are discussed in detail in subsequent chapters.

Substance Abuse

The list of substances ingested, smoked, or "snorted" by people is disturbingly long. Whenever possible, patients who care about vocal quality should be educated by their physicians about the deleterious effects of such habits on their voices and the longevity of their careers. The harmful effects of tobacco smoke on mucosa are indisputable. It causes erythema, edema, and generalized inflammation throughout the vocal tract. Marijuana produces a particularly irritating, unfiltered smoke, which is inhaled directly, causing considerable mucosal response.

Smoking should not be permitted in the serious singer or actor. Performers who are required to perform in smoke-filled environments may suffer from the same effects from second-hand smoke. In some situations, this may be made less troublesome by placing a quiet fan behind the singer or speaker to direct the smoke out toward the audience and away from the stage and by limiting the periods of exposure.

A history of alcohol abuse suggests the probability of poor vocal technique. Intoxication results in muscular incoordination and decreased sensory awareness which undermine vocal discipline designed to optimize and protect the voice. The medical effect of *small* amounts of alcohol is controversial. Although many experts oppose it because of its vasodilation and consequent mucosal alteration, many people do not seem to be adversely affected by limited quantities of alcohol, such as a glass of wine with dinner, preceding a performance. However, patients should be able to identify and avoid specific types of wine or beer that cause nasal congestion or rhinorrhea (nasal drainage). Food allergies to these substances are common and may interfere with vocal performance.

Benzodiazepines, barbiturates, narcotics, alcohol, and chronic use of all other drugs that alter sensorium or fine motor control should also be prohibited in serious voice users. Central nervous system depressants should be used only as prescribed, for short periods and specific medical indications. They have potential for tolerance, dependence, and "self-medication" for mood disorders.

Cocaine use is increasingly common, especially among pop musicians. It can be extremely irritating to the nasal mucosa, causes marked vasoconstriction, and may alter sensorium, resulting in decreased voice control and a tendency to vocal abuse. In addition, small amounts of cocaine may reach the larynx, resulting in vocal fold anesthesia and predisposing the vocalist to serious injury. The psychological and social consequences of cocaine abuse are well known to psychological professionals.

Patients, especially performers, frequently borrow drugs from each other and may unwittingly abuse prescription medications, as well. Antihistamines, antibiotics, and diuretics are the most commonly abused agents. Patients usually know better and are reluctant to admit to this behavior; so the question must be asked specifically by the physician during acquisition of the medical history.

MEMBERS OF THE VOICE TREATMENT TEAM

Medical management of many problems affecting the voice involves voice therapy which is provided in an interdisciplinary fashion. The role and training of each of these specialists is described so that the psychotherapist may participate knowledgeably in this team approach.

The Speech-Language Pathologist

An excellent speech-language pathologist is invaluable in the care of patients with vocal complaints. Like physicians and most other medical professionals, speech-language pathologists have varied backgrounds, experience, and interest areas. In fact, most speech-language pathology programs teach relatively little about caring for professional speakers and nothing about professional singers. Moreover, few speech-language pathologists have vast clinical experience in this specialized area, and there are as yet no fellowships in this specialty for speech-language pathologists. Speech-language pathologists often subspecialize. A person who expertly treats patients for neurologic consequences following a CVA, provides voice rehabilitation after laryngectomy, treats stuttering, or manages swallowing disorders may not necessarily know how to manage professional voice users optimally.

Laryngologists who refer voice patients to independent clinicians for therapy must learn the strengths and weaknesses of the speech-language pathologists with whom they work. Once a speech-language pathologist who is interested in treating professional voice users is identified, the laryngologist and speech-language pathologist should work together closely as a collaborative team. In general, therapy should be directed toward relaxation techniques, breath control, and abdominal support. Patients who seek voice care at centers specializing in Performing Arts Medicine will usually obtain this level of expert care. Another source of education and medical referral is The Voice Foundation (1721 Pine Street, Philadelphia, PA 19103).

Voice therapy may be helpful even for singers who have no obvious problem with the speaking voice, but who have significant technical problems with singing. Once a person has been singing for several years, it is often difficult for a singing teacher to convince him or her to correct certain habitual technical errors. Singers are much less guarded about their speaking voices. Therefore, a speech-language pathologist may be able to rapidly teach proper breath support, relaxation, and voice placement in speaking. Once they are mastered, these techniques can be carried over fairly easily into singing through cooperative efforts of the speech-language pathologist and the singing teacher.

This "back door" approach has proven extremely useful in our center.[1] For the actor, it is often helpful to coordinate speech-language pathology sessions with acting-voice training, and especially with the personalized training of the "stage speaking voice" provided by the actor's voice teacher or coach. Information provided by the speech-language pathologist, the acting-voice trainer, and the singing teacher should be symbiotic and should not conflict. This requires timely, open communication among these professionals. If there are major discrepancies, misunderstanding of the instructions by the patient or an improper training suggestion from one of the team members should be suspected, and discussion leading to the appropriate changes should occur promptly.[1]

Singing Teachers

In selected patients, singing lessons may also be extremely helpful, even in nonsingers with voice problems. The training techniques used to develop abdominothoracic strength, breath control, laryngeal and neck muscle strength, and relaxation are very similar to those used in speech therapy. Singing lessons often expedite voice therapy and appear to improve the end result in some patients.

A small group of specially trained singing teachers called "singing voice specialists" has emerged.[1] They have acquired extra interdisciplinary knowledge and skills needed to work effectively with patients who have vocal fold injuries. Because the voice and singing are so personal, a fairly trusting, intimate clinical relationship commonly develops quickly in the voice studio; and patients often reveal information to singing voice specialists that they found difficult to discuss with the laryngologist or even the speech-language pathologist. Singing voice specialists are often the members of the voice team who first recognize the need for psychological assessment and treatment, especially in centers where the Arts Medicine psychologist sees patients only on referral.

Acting-Voice Trainer

The use of acting-voice trainers (drama voice coaches) as members of the medical team is new.[1] This addition to the team has been extremely valuable to patients and other team members. Like singing voice specialists, professionals with education in theater arts utilize numerous vocal and body movement techniques that not only enhance physical function, but also release tension and break down emotional barriers that may impede optimal voice function. Tearful revelations to the acting-voice trainer are not uncommon; and, like the singing teacher, this individual may identify psychological and emotional problems interfering with professional success that have been skillfully hidden from other professionals on the voice team and in the patient's life.

CONCLUSION

Many diagnoses and treatments are important in caring for voice patients. Those discussed in this chapter are among the most common. The exacting demands of a professional singer or actor, his or her acute ability to analyze the body's condition, and his or her professional athlete's need for a nearly perfect treatment result provide special challenges and gratification for physicians, psychological professionals, speech-language pathologists, and other healthcare providers. However, a great many voice patients who are not performers are also extremely dependent on voice quality and endurance for career advancement. Consequently, every patient with a voice complaint should be treated as Luciano Pavarotti, James Earl Jones, or Barbra Streisand would be treated; and every voice evaluation should be carried out systematically until a diagnosis has been made on the basis of positive medical evidence. The emergence of interdisciplinary teams, advanced instrumentation, and voice laboratories has led to dramatic improvements in the standard of voice care. The rapid development of voice as a subspecialty promises continuing advances in the care of voice disorders. The availability of psychological professionals who subspecialize in patients with voice dysfunction has added an additional dimension to the care and comfort of these complex patients.

REFERENCES

1. Sataloff RT. *Professional Voice: The Science and Art of Clinical Care*, 2nd ed. San Diego, Calif: Singular Publishing Group Inc; 1997.
2. Abitbol J. Limitations of the laser in microsurgery of the larynx. In: Lawrence VL, ed. *Transactions of the Twelfth Symposium: Care of the Professional Voice.* New York, NY: The Voice Foundation; 1984:297-301.
3. Tapia RG, Pardo J, Marigil M, Pacio A. Effects of the laser upon Reinke's space and the neural system of the vocalis muscle. In: Lawrence VL, ed. *Transactions of the Twelfth Symposium: Care of the Professional Voice.* New York, NY: The Voice Foundation; 1984:289-291.
4. Spiegel JR, Sataloff RT, Cohn JR, et al. Respiratory function in singer: medical assessment, diagnoses, and treatments. *J Voice.* 1988;2(1):40-50.
5. Spiegel J, Sataloff RT. *Voice Surgery.* St. Louis, Mo: Mosby Year-Book Inc; 1993.
6. Arndt, HJ. Stimmstorungen nach Behandlung mit androgenen und anabolen Hormonen. *Munch Med Wochenschr.* 1974;116:1715-1720.
7. Bourdial, J. Les troubles de la voix provoques par la therapeutique hormonale androgene. *Ann Otolaryngol* (Paris). 1970;87:725-734.
8. Ackerman, R, Pfan W. Gerotologische Untersuchungen zur Storunepanfalligkeit der Sprechstimme bei Berufssprechern. *Folia Phoniat.* 1974;25:95-99.
9. von Leden H. Speech and hearing problems in the geriatric patient. *J Am Geriat Soc.* 1977;25:422-426.
10. Rubin J, Sataloff RT, Korovin G, Gould WJ. *The Diagnosis and Treatment of Voice Disorders.* New York, NY: Igaku-Shoin Medical Publishers Inc; 1995.
11. Gupta OP, Bhatia PL, Agarwal MK, Mehrotra ML, Mishr SK. Nasal pharyngeal and laryngeal manifestations of hypothyroidism. *Ear, Nose and Throat.* 1977;56(9):10-21.
12. Punt NA. Applied laryngology—singers and actors. *Proc R Soc Med.* 1968;61:1152-1156.
13. Ritter RN. The effect of hypothyroidism on the larynx of the rat. *Ann Otol Rhinol Laryngol.* 1964;67:404-416.
14. Malinsky M, et al. Étude clinique et electrophysiologique des alterations de la voix au cours des thyrotoxioses. *Ann Endocrinol* (Paris). 1977;38:171-172.
15. Lacina V. Der Einfluss der Menstruation auf die Stimme der Sangerinnen. *Folia Phoniat.* 1968;20:13-24.
16. Wendler J. Zyklusabhangige Leistungsschwankungen der Stimme und ihre Beeinflussung durch Ovulationshemmer. *Folia Phoniat* (Basel). 1972;24(4):259-277.
17. Brodnitz F. Medical care preventive therapy (panel). In: Lawrence V, ed. *Transcripts of the Seventh Annual Symposium: Care of the Professional Voice.* New York, NY: The Voice Foundation. 1978;3:86.
18. Dordain M. Étude statistique de l'influence des contraceptifs hormonaux sur la voix. *Folia Phoniat.* 1972;24:86-96.
19. Pahn V, Goretzlehner G. Stimmstorungen durch hormonale Kontrazeptiva. *Zentralb Gynakol.* 1978;100:341-346.

20. Schiff M. "The pill" in otolaryngology. *Trans Am Acad Ophthalmol Otolaryngol.* 1968;72:76-84.
21. Deuster CV. Irreversible Stimmstorung in der Schwangerscheft. *HNO.* 1977;25:430-432.
22. Flach M, Schwickardi H, Simen R. Welchen Einfluss haben Menstruation and Schwangerschaft auf die augsgebildete Gesangsstimme? *Folia Phonat.* 1968;21:199-210.
23. Damste PH. Virilization of the voice due to anabolic steroids. *Folia Phoniat.* 1964;16:10-18.
24. Damste PH. Voice changes in adult women caused by virilizing agents. *J Speech Hear Disord.* 1967;32:126-132.
25. Gates GA, Saegert J, Wilson N, Johnson L, Sheperd A, Hearnd EM. Effects of beta-blockade on singing performance. *Ann Otol Rhinol Laryngol.* 1985;94:570-574.
26. Saez S, Francoise S. Recepteurs d'androgenes: mise en evidence dans la fraction cytosolique de muqueuse normale et d'epitheliomas pharyngolarynges humains. *CR Acad Sci* (Paris). 1975;280:935-938.
27. Vuorenkoski V, Lenko HL, Tjernlund P, Vuorenkoski L, Perheentupa J. Fundamental voice frequency during normal and abnormal growth, and after androgen treatment. *Arch Dis Child.* 1978;53:201-209.

CHAPTER

5

General and Psychotropic Medications and Their Effects on the Voice

Psychotherapists work constantly with patients who ingest drugs. In some cases, they are common, "socially acceptable" chemicals such as alcohol, nicotine, and caffeine. In other cases, they are illegal, unacceptable drugs such as crack-cocaine. In either instance, most psychological professionals know intuitively that there are hazards associated with the use of such substances. However, the risks associated with commonly prescribed medications, and even routine over-the-counter medications like aspirin, may be less apparent. It is extremely important for clinicians to be familiar with the potential vocal risks of drug use and to teach their patients to be informed consumers.

Virtually all medications have some laryngeal effect. In many instances, the effects are clinically insignificant. However, some common medications have a significant impact upon the voice, and all voice professionals should be familiar with drug-induced phenomena that may alter vocal function. This important subject is discussed at length elsewhere,[1,2] but many of the most important aspects are highlighted in this chapter.

Antibiotics

Antibiotics are commonly used to treat bacterial infections. Ideally, antibiotic selection is guided by culture result. However, more commonly, antibiotics are prescribed empirically. Inappropriate antibiotic prescription may damage the voice by allowing progression of a potentially curable infection. However, even appropriate antibiotics have potential side effects that may alter the voice. These include allergy, dryness, metallic taste, and secondary yeast infections among others.

Anti-Viral Agents

A few anti-viral agents are now available. Acyclovir is used specifically for herpes and may be appropriate in patients with herpetic recurrent superior laryngeal nerve paralysis. Amantadine appears useful against influenza A.[3-6] It may also have some beneficial effects against other viruses. If a performer must work in an area in which there is a flu epidemic, it may be reasonable to use this drug. However, agitation, tachycardia, and extreme xerostomia and xerophonia (dry mouth and voice) may occur. When these side effects are present, they are generally severe enough to require cancellation of a performance.

Antihistamines

Normal phonation requires uninhibited movement of the vibratory margin of the vocal folds, and normal mucosal secretions are exceedingly important. If vocal tract lubrication is impaired, aberrations in phonation occur. When singers or public speakers develop thick, viscous vocal fold secretions during performance, the effects can be catastrophic. Excessive drying of the upper respiratory tract is the vocal complication associated with the largest number of medications, and it is especially prominent following antihistamine ingestion.

Antihistamines may be used to treat allergies. However, virtually all antihistamines can exert a drying effect on upper respiratory tract secretions, although severity varies widely from drug to drug and from person to person. In addition, antihistamines are often combined with sympathomimetic or parasympatholytic agents which further reduce and thicken mucosal secretion and may reduce lubrication to the point of producing a dry cough. This may be more harmful to phonation than the allergic condition itself. Often the patient has self-medicated with an over-the-counter (OTC) antihistamine preparation. The majority of antihistamine agents are acetylcholine antagonists, and this parasympatholytic activity probably accounts for the increased viscosity of secretions. Interestingly, antihistamines used to treat allergies do not act to block the stimulant effects of histamine on gastric acid secretions, but do affect salivary glands and mucous-secreting membranes of the respiratory tract. They may also have sedative effects which impair sensorium and disturb performance. These are distinct from the effects achieved by chemically different antihistamines used to treat other conditions such as reflux (cimetidine, ranitidine, and other H_2 blockers).[2]

Mucolytic and Wetting Agents

The viscosity of upper respiratory tract secretions is affected significantly by environmental dryness. Feder[7] has described the drying effects of airplane flight and the resultant irritation of respiratory tract mucosa. Similar problems occur when mountain climbing or traveling to cities located at high altitudes. The coaching staffs of athletic teams have long been aware of the deleterious effects of dehydration on general body function. These well-known factors may impinge on the vocal professional as a result of recreational practices, such as jogging, especially if done in hot or dry environments, or as a consequence of strenuous rehearsal and performance.

The viscosity of upper respiratory secretions is directly related to the availability of body water, assuming that no metabolic or pharmacologic agents have been interposed. The ideal wetting agent for respiratory tract secretions is water in the form of increased fluid intake and an elevated environmental humidity. Other wetting agents often used for dryness of respiratory tract secretions are expectorants or mucolytics. Although these agents are less effective than water and subject to individual variation, dry mucous membranes will usually respond favorably. Entex (Baylor) is a useful expectorant and vasoconstrictor that increases and thins mucosal secretions. Guaifenesin also thins and increases secretions. Humibid (Adams) is currently among the most convenient preparations available. These drugs are relatively harmless and may be very helpful in singers who complain of thick secretions, frequent throat clearing, or "postnasal drip." Awareness of postnasal drip is often caused by secretions that are too thick rather than too plentiful.

Diuretics and Other Nonsteriod Medications for Edema

Transudation of body water from the vascular system producing edema and subsequent swelling of soft tissues of the respiratory tract is a commonly encountered phenomenon. Physical trauma to the mucous membranes, which occurs with inappropriate voice use or abuse, is frequently etiologic in vocal fold edema. In response to a variety of stimuli, water leaves the circulatory system and enters the submucosal spaces of the vocal tract, including areas in the vocal folds and the air passages themselves. Under most circumstances, edema of the vocal folds will be caused by protein-bound water.[8] As such, it will not be ameliorated by diuretic agents commonly prescribed for tissue edema. Diuretic use for premenstrual voice change is common but inappropriate because it does not alleviate protein-bound edema in Reinke's space, but does produce undesirable dehydration.[2] Voice patients using diuretics for any disease condition (such as hypertension) must be monitored closely for adverse effects of diuretics caused by drying.

Decongestants

Another group of pharmacological agents used for soft tissue edema in the respiratory tract includes the topical or systemic decongestants. Their primary action involves reduction in the diameter and volume of vascular structures in the submucosal area, but they may also produce "rebound" dilatation and edema. These decongestants include norepinephrine used as an inhalant and pseudoephedrine. Effects of sprays are discussed below.

Corticosteroids

Corticosteroids are extremely effective anti-inflammatory agents and may be prescribed for the management of acute inflammatory laryngitis. Occasionally, they also may be appropriate for use in infectious laryngitis when extraordinary performance obligations supervene. Appropriate steroid dosing is controversial. Additional study is necessary to establish valid recommendations. Care must be taken not to prescribe steroids indiscriminately. They should be used only when the physician determines that there is a pressing, professional voice commitment that is being hampered by vocal fold inflammation. If an infectious origin is suspected, antibiotic coverage is recommended.

Corticosteroids may have adverse effects. Although such effects are not generally seen following the short-term steroid use appropriate for an acute voice problem, they may occur in any patient. The more common corticosteroid side effects include gastric irritation with possible ulceration and hemorrhage, insomnia, mild mucosal drying, mood change (euphoria, occasionally psychosis), and irritability. Long-term effects such as muscle wasting and fat redistribution generally are not encountered following appropriate short-term use of steroids. Corticosteroids in high dose or for prolonged periods may also be required in patients with other concomitant diseases such as severe asthma or a number of autoimmune diseases. Prolonged dosing may lead to significant side effects such as cataracts, glaucoma, hypertension, susceptibility to infection, gastric ulceration, risk of pulmonary embolus, Cushing's syndrome, and thinning and fragility of skin and bones.[9(p45)]

Another potential problem peculiar to professional voice users is steroid abuse. Because side effects are uncommon and steroids work extremely well, there is a tendency (especially among singers) to overuse or abuse them. This practice must be avoided.

Sprays, Mists, and Inhalants

Diphenhydramine hydrochloride (Benadryl [Parke-Davis]), 0.5 percent in distilled water, delivered to the larynx as a mist may be helpful for its vasoconstrictive properties, but it is also dangerous because of its analgesic effect. However, Punt has advocated use of this mixture and several modifications of it.[10] Other topical vasoconstrictors that do not contain analgesics may be prescribed in selected cases. Oxymetazoline hydrochloride (Afrin [Schering]) applied by large particle mist to the larynx is particularly helpful in treating severe edema immediately prior to performance, but it should be used *only* by the physician under emergent, extreme circumstances. Five percent propylene glycol in a physiologically balanced salt solution may be delivered by large particle mist and can provide helpful lubrication, particularly in cases of laryngitis sicca following air travel or associated with dry climates.[2] Such treatment is harmless and may also provide a beneficial placebo effect. Water, saline, or other balanced fluid delivered via a vaporizer or steam generator is frequently effective and sufficient. This therapy should be augmented by oral hydration which is the mainstay of treatment for dehydration. A patient can monitor his or her state of hydration by observing urine color. Patients will be instructed to "pee pale."

Nasal medications such as Beconase (Allen & Hanburys), Vancenase (Schering), and Nasacort (Rhône-Poulenc Rorer) do not seem to harm the voice. However, most inhalers are not recommended for use in professional voice users. Many people develop contact inflammation from sensitivity to the propellants used in inhalers; and propellants may also cause mucosal drying. Steroid inhalers used for prolonged periods may also result in candida laryngitis. In addition, dysphonia occurs in up to 50% of patients using steroid inhalers, related to the aerosolized steroid itself and not to the Freon propellant.[11] Prolonged inhaled steroid use, such as is common in asthmatics, also may capable of causing wasting of the vocalis muscle.

Antitussive Medications

Cough suppressant mixtures, especially preparations containing codeine,[12] often include agents that have a secondary drying effect on vocal tract secretions.[13] Antihistamines are also common ingredients in antitussives. Dextromethorphan has pharmacologic effects similar to those of codeine and is encountered in a variety of OTC preparations. Generally, preparations that contain dextromethorphan and a wetting agent such as guaifenesin work well for voice patients.

Antihypertensive Agents

Almost all of the current antihypertensive agents have some degree of parasympathomimetic effect and thus dry mucous membranes of the upper respiratory tract. They commonly are used in combination with diuretic agents that also promote dehydration.[12] In some circumstances, the laryngologist may find this drying effect substantial enough to merit recommending that the patient's internist prescribe another antihypertensive agent. Among the more troublesome drugs are reserpines and agents of the methyldopa group. Coughing is a side effect of some of these medications, and their use should be considered in the differential diagnosis of patients with nonproductive, irritative cough.

Gastroenterologic Medications

Antispasmodic agents are well known for their ability to reduce pain and motility arising from smooth muscles, especially those of the gastrointestinal tract. H_2 blockers and proton pump inhibitors, which decrease the amount of stomach acid formed, have revolutionized the treatment of gastric ulcers and have proven very useful in laryngology for the treatment of gastroesophageal reflux laryngitis. Although drying of the laryngeal mucosa is not a major side effect of the H_2 blockers, it does occur and must be considered.[2] Other gastric medications include phenobarbital, prochlorperazine, isopropamide, and propantheline bromide. Members of the belladonna alkaloid group including scopolamine and atropine are widely used and prescribed for their antispasmodic effects. All of these agents have significant drying effects on secretions in the vocal tract.[12]

Vitamin C

Not infrequently, the laryngologist encounters a patient who consumes large amounts of vitamin C (ascorbic acid) in an effort to maintain health or to prevent the occurrence of a common cold. In some patients, a drying effect similar to that of a mild antihistamine occurs when vitamin C is taken in large doses.[14,15] Additionally, a patient with less than optimal renal function may produce acid urine and possibly form renal calculi (kidney stones).

Sleeping Pills

Sleeping pills should be used with great caution. Many of them cause alterations in sensorium and dryness which may affect the voice adversely especially early in the day following use. Others cause rebound insomnia and/or confusion. They also have the potential for tolerance and addiction.

Analgesics

Aspirin and other analgesics frequently are prescribed for relief of minor throat and laryngeal irritation. The platelet dysfunction caused by aspirin predisposes to hemorrhage, especially in vocal folds traumatized by excessive voice use in the face of vocal dysfunction. Mucosal hemorrhage can be devastating to a professional voice user, and aspirin products should be avoided altogether in singers. Acetaminophen is the best substitute, as even the most common nonsteroidal anti-inflammatory drugs such as ibuprofen may interfere with the clotting mechanism. Caruso reportedly used a spray of ether and iodoform on his vocal folds when he had to sing with laryngitis. Nevertheless, the use of analgesics is extremely dangerous and should be avoided. Pain is an important protective physiologic function. Masking it risks incurring significant vocal damage that may be unrecognized until after the analgesic or anesthetic wears off.

Hormones

Hormone medications may cause substantial changes in voice quality due to alterations in fluid content or structural changes. Structural alterations in laryngeal architecture seldom occur as the result of pharmacologic influences, but androgens are an exception. They may produce permanent lowering of the fundamental frequencies, especially in females, and coarsening of the voice.[17-22] Androgenic agents frequently are used in the treatment of endometriosis and as part of chemotherapy regimens for breast cancer. Professional voice users especially should be informed of potential voice changes before these medications are employed, and their use should be avoided whenever possible.

Birth control pills with relatively high progesterone content are most likely to produce androgen-like changes in the voice. Most oral contraceptives marketed in the last several years have had appropriate estrogen-progesterone balance, and voice changes are seen in only about 5% of women who use birth control pills.[23-31] These changes generally are temporary, abating when oral contraceptive use is discontinued. Estrogen replacement is helpful in forestalling the typical voice changes that follow menopause. Sequential hormone replacement is most physiologic. Unless medical contraindications are present, women concerned about voice preservation should discuss hormone replacement under appropriate medical supervision at the time of menopause.

Other endocrine medications also may affect the voice, often beneficially. Thyroid replacement may restore vocal efficiency and "ring" lost with even a mild degree of hypothyroidism. Agents used to treat maladies in any part of the diencephalic-pituitary axis should be presumed to have laryngeal effects and warrant close monitoring of voice function.

Broncho-Active Medications

Optimal vocal function depends on the availability of a powerfully supported air stream passing between the vocal folds. Impairment of pulmonary function can cause severe problems for professional voice users. Pulmonary function is affected deleteriously by bronchoconstricting agents. Bronchodilators are often helpful, especially for patients with reactive airway disease, although inhaled bronchodilators may produce laryngitis, as discussed above in the section on other inhalers. Clinically, inhaled cromolyn sodium appears to cause fewer problems than most of the other agents commonly used in the treatment of asthma. The most commonly used bronchodilator is epinephrine and its related compounds, including xanthines (aminophylline is an example).[2] They can be used to counter the bronchoconstrictive effects of environmental factors such as house dust, pollen, other allergenic agents, and common air pollutants produced by our increasingly industrialized society. Active bronchoconstriction occurs in allergic reactions and in asthma. These conditions may seriously hamper or prevent vocal performance unless recognized and treated properly.

NEUROLOGIC MEDICATIONS

Professional voice users may be diagnosed with neurologic disease entities either in the course of the evaluation of their voice complaint or as a co-existing illness (see Chapter 12). A number of highly potent medications are available for use in a medical treatment regimen. The side effects of the medication or the course of the illness itself may necessitate performance modifications or ultimately force the end of a performance career. Physicians and other health care providers should be especially familiar with a few of the most common illnesses and the usual medications prescribed.

Parkinson's disease may be treated by anticholinergic agents, L-dopa (and L-dopa in combination with other agents), dopamine receptor agonists, amantadine hydrochloride, and MAO-inhibitors. Side effects are related to the drug's mechanisms of action in the central nervous system and peripheral target organs.[9(p29-135)] Anticholinergic side effects include blurred vision, dryness, impaired urination, constipation, nervousness, dizziness, drowsiness, headache, confusion, memory loss, hallucination, and delusions.[31] The side effects most commonly associated with L-dopa are GI disturbance, orthostatic hypotension, syncope, oral dryness, blurred vision, and cardiac arrhythmias. Dyskinesias, nightmares, confusion, agitation, psychosis, depression, increased libido, and end-of-dose akinesia have also been also reported.[9(p29-135)] L-dopa is sometimes given in a drug combination to decrease peripheral systemic side effects.

Amantadine, another drug for Parkinson's disease, has side effects similar to the anticholinergics. Dopamine receptor agonists produce GI disturbance, postural hypotension, and fatigue, as well as skin rash, headache, involuntary movements, depression, and sometimes confusion or hallucinations.[9(p29-135)] The side effects of monamine oxidase inhibitors are described in detail in the section on psychoactive drugs. Parkinsonian syndromes not secondary to Parkinson's disease may also be a focus of treatment with these drugs.

Myasthenia gravis is an autoimmune disease in which blood antibodies impair synaptic transmission at the neuromuscular junction by disturbance of the neurotransmitter acetylcholine. Drugs are used to treat myasthenia gravis by enhancing the action of acetylcholine (by inhibiting acetylcholinesterase) or by immune suppression. Acetylcholinesterase inhibitors most commonly cause side effects of excessive salivation or GI disturbances. Skin, rash, nervousness, confusion, or weakness have also been reported.[9(p29-135)] Corticosteroid side effects were described previously. Other immunosuppressants may also be used in patients with an inability to tolerate corticosteroids, but they have side effects that may be extremely serious.

Multiple sclerosis involves the progressive loss of myelin in white matter adjacent to the ventricles and in the optic nerves, brain stem, cerebellum, spinal cord, and elsewhere in the central nervous system. Drug therapy aims at reducing the frequency of exacerbations and/or reducing the degree of myelin loss. Medications include immunosuppressants such as corticosteroids, adrenocorticotropic hormone, azathioprine, and cyclophosphamide. The most common side effects of immunosuppression have been discussed. Beta-interferon side effects include local inflammation and flulike syndrome.[9(p29-135)] Medications also are used to treat associated symptoms such as spasticity, cerebellar dysfunction, and depression.

Beta-Blockers

Within the last few years, propranolol and other beta-blockers have been designated in the literature as useful for stage fright. Although British investigators[31] reported that instrumental musicians given this potent beta-blocker did, in fact, exhibit less anxiety during performance, a unanimous response in voice professionals was not seen.

A subsequent study appears to indicate that propranolol, given for preperformance anxiety, lessened anxiety, and also produced an increase in salivation.[32] This investigation was conducted by measuring the weight increase in saliva-saturated dental rolls of cotton placed in the mouth during performance. This indicated that the problem of upper respiratory tract secretion dryness had been avoided and that some of the parasympathomimetic effects of performance anxiety had been negated. The laryngologic community generally agrees that these drugs should not be used for singers.

They are potentially dangerous, affecting heart rate, blood pressure, and provoking asthma attacks in susceptible patients. In addition, when given in doses sufficient to ameliorate stage fright, they produce a lackluster performance.[33] Moreover, any professional voice user who requires an ingested substance to perform the daily activities or his or her chosen profession is revealing a significant problem. Physicians should refer such a patient for appropriate counseling and treatment of the *cause* of the problem, not merely medicate the symptom.

Central Nervous System Stimulants

Central nervous system stimulants, such as cocaine, amphetamines, "diet pills," and other vasoconstrictor agents are to be regarded skeptically. An idiosyncratic response to a vasoconstrictor, such as a pseudoephedrine, or an overdose of such an OTC medication may manifest itself as acute central nervous system stimulation. Added to the "adrenalin high" of performance in the actor or musical performer, the combination of effects may very well be deleterious.

Central Nervous System Depressants

Use of central nervous system depressants is also questionable in people who use their voices in a competitive way. In this category are alcohol, barbiturates, sedative-hypnotics, and marijuana. Alteration of sensory input either by a stimulant or a depressant is potentially hazardous in a voice professional. The patient who is unaware of these effects should be apprised of them promptly by the laryngologist.

PSYCHOACTIVE MEDICATIONS

All psychoactive agents have effects that can interfere with vocal tract physiology. Treatment requires frequent, open collaboration between the laryngologist and the psychiatrist specializing in psychopharmacology. The patient and physicians need to carefully weigh the benefits and side effects of available medications. Patients must be informed of the relative probability of experiencing any known side effect. This is especially critical to the professional voice user and will play an important role in developing a treatment plan in which there is no imminent serious psychiatric risk.

Antidepressant medications include compounds from several different classes. Tri- and tetracyclic antidepressants (TCAs) block the reuptake of norepinephrine and serotonin and have secondary effects on pre- and postsynaptic receptors. H_1 and H_2 receptor blockade has also been demonstrated.[34] These drugs include imipramine hydrochloride (Tofranil), trimipramine maleate (Sermontil), amitriptyline (Elavil), doxepine hydrochloride (Sinequan), desipramine (Norpramine), protriptyline (Vivactil), and nortriptyline hydrochloride (Pamelor).[9(p29-135),34]

Schatzberg and Cole summarized the side effects of TCAs as *anticholinergic* (dry mouth and nasal mucosa, constipation, urinary hesitancy, gastroesophageal reflux), *autonomic* (orthostatic hypotension, palpitations, increased cardiac conduction intervals, diaphoresis, hypertension, tremor), *allergic* (skin rashes), *CNS* (stimulation, sedation, delirium, twitching, nausea, speech delay, seizures, extrapyramidal symptoms), and *other* (weight gain, impotence). These may be dose-related and agent specific.[34]

Monamine oxidase inhibitors (MAOIs) are useful in treating depression that is refractory to tricyclics. The mode of action involves inhibiting monoamine oxidase in various organs, especially MAO-A for which norepinephrine and serotonin are primary substrates. The full restoration of enzyme activity may require 2 weeks after the drug is discontinued. The most commonly prescribed MAOIs are phenelzine (Nardil), tranylcypromine (Parnate), and isocarboxazid (Marplan).[34]

The side effects of MAOIs may be extremely serious and troublesome. The one most commonly reported is dizziness secondary to orthostatic hypotension. When taking MAOIs, hypertensive crisis with

violent headache and potential CVA, or hyperpyrexic crisis with mono-
clonus and coma, may be produced by ingesting foods rich in tyramine
and many medications. These include Demerol, epinephrine, local
anesthetics containing sympathomimetics, decongestants, surgical
anesthetics, and nasal sprays. Patients for whom these medications are
prescribed must be carefully instructed and ordinarily sign informed
consent indicating that they understand the potential drug and food interactions. They must carefully monitor their diets. Other side effects
include sexual dysfunction, sedation, insomnia, overstimulation,
myositislike reactions, myoclonic twitches, and a small incidence of dry
mouth, constipation, and urinary hesitancy.[9(p29-135),34-36]

A few antidepressants have been developed with different chemical
structures and side effect profiles. Trazodone (Desyrel) is a pharmacologically complex agent which blocks 5-HT_2 receptors and inhibits 5-HT
reuptake. It is not as potent a reuptake inhibitor as fluoxetine, serataline,
or paroxetine.[36] It has proven helpful in depression associated with initial insomnia. The side effects are particularly noteworthy: sedation,
acute dizziness with fainting (especially when taken on an empty stomach), gastrointestinal disturbance, blurred vision, dry mouth, extrapyramidal symptoms, arrhythmias, leukopenia, and priapism.[9(p29-135),34]

Bupropion (Wellbutrin) was released in 1989. Its biochemical mode
of action is not well understood. It is neither an uptake inhibitor nor a
MAOI. Its probable mode of action is on the dopamine mechanism. The
most commonly reported complaint is nausea. However, a potential risk
of seizures exists, and the drug is not recommended in patients with a
history of seizure, head trauma, or anorexia/bulimia.[34,35] Nefazodone
(Serzone) shares side effects with other antidepressants. Notable drug
interactions may be problematic in professional voice users because this
drug should not be taken with triazolam (Halcion), alprazolam (Xanax),
terfanadine (Seldane), astemizole (Hismanal), or cisipride (Propulsid).[37]

A smaller group of antidepressant drugs which selectively inhibit
the reuptake of serotonin are most likely to be selected as first pharmacologic agents. These include fluoxetine (Prozac), serataline (Zoloft),
and paroxetine (Paxil). They appear to be effective in typical episodic
depression and for some chronic refractory presentations.[36,39] Major
side effects are significant degrees of nausea, sweating, headache,
mouth dryness, tremor, nervousness, dizziness, insomnia, somnolence,
constipation, and sexual dysfunction, although the relative incidence of
these varies from agent to agent. Venlafaxine hydrochloride (Effexor) is
a reuptake inhibitor of serotonin, norepinephrine, and, weakly,
dopamine. Its major side effect is sustained hypertension which is partially dose-dependent.[38,39] There are drug interactions with concomi-

tant administration of tryptophan, MAOIs, warfarin, cimetidine, phenobarbital, and phenytoin.[38,39]

"Mood stabilizing" drugs are effective in manic episodes and prevent manic and depressive recurrences in patients with bipolar disorder. These include lithium salts and several anticonvulsants. Lithium is available in multiple formulations and prescribing is guided by both symptom index and blood levels. Lithium side effects are apparent in diverse organ systems. The most commonly noted is fine tremor, especially noticeable in the fingers. With toxic lithium levels, gross tremulousness, ataxia, dysarthria, and confusion or delirium may develop. Some patients describe slowed mentation, measurable memory deficit, and "impaired creativity." Chronic nausea and diarrhea are usually related to GI tract mucosal irritation, but may be signs of toxicity. Some patients gain weight progressively and may demonstrate edema or increased appetite. Lithium therapy affects thyroid function. In some cases it is transitory, but there may be goiter with normal T_3 and T_4, but elevated TSH. Undesirable effects of carbamazepine include serious adverse consequences such as severe dermatitis, stomatis, lymphadenopathy, renal damage, depression and agitation, diplopia, peripheral neuritis, and potential thrombophlebitis. Latent psychosis and systemic lupus erythematosus have been reported to be activated by use of this drug. More minor complications include headache, dizziness or vertigo, drowsiness, ataxia, visual blurring, tinnitus, appetite and gastrointestinal disturbances, edema, changes in skin pigmentation, alopecia, and aching discomfort in the muscles and joints.[9(p 29-135),34]

Polyuria and secondary polydipsia are complications of lithium and may progress to diabetes insipidus. In most cases, discontinuing the medication reverses the renal effects. Prescribed thiazide diuretics can double the lithium level and lead to sudden lithium toxicity. Nonsteroidal anti-inflammatory drugs decrease lithium excretion. Cardiovascular effects include the rare induction of "sick sinus syndrome." Aggravation of psoriasis, allergic skin rashes, and reversible alopecia are associated with lithium therapy, as are teratogenic effects.[34]

Three anticonvulsant compounds appear to act preferentially on the temporal lobe and the limbic system. Carbamazepine (Tegretol) carries a risk of agranulocytosis or aplastic anemia, and it is monitored by CBC and symptoms of bone marrow depression. Care must be taken to avoid the numerous drug interactions which accelerate the metabolism of some drugs or raise carbamazepine levels.[34]

Valproic acid (Depakote, Depakene) is especially useful where there is a "rapid cycling" pattern. The major side effect is a risk of hepatocellular toxicity. Thrombocytopenia and platelet dysfunction have been reported. Sedation is common and tremor, ataxia, weight gain, alopecia, and fetal neural tube defects are all side effects which patients must comprehend.[34]

Anxiolytics are the most commonly prescribed psychotropic drugs, usually by nonpsychiatric specialists for somatic disorders. It behooves the laryngologist and mental health provider to probe for a history of past or current drug therapy in markedly anxious or somatically focused patients with vocal complaints. Commonly prescribed benzodiazepines include: alprazolam (Xanax), chlordiazepoxide hydrochloride (Librium), clorazepate dipotassium (Tranxene), diazepam (Valium), lorazepam (Ativan), oxazepam (Serax), and clonazepam (Klonopin). Benzodiazepines produce effective relief of anxiety, but have a high addictive potential which includes physical symptoms of withdrawal, including potential seizures, if the drug is stopped abruptly. The most common benzodiazepine side effect is dose-related sedation, followed by dizziness, weakness, ataxia, decreased motor performance, and mild hypotension.[34] Clonazepam (Klonopin) is a benzodiazepine and may also produce malcoordination as well as disinhibition, agitation, or asituational anger.[9(p29-135),34] Alterations of sensory input, either by CNS stimulants (cocaine, amphetamines, and OTC vasoconstrictors) or depressants, are potentially dangerous in a voice professional. An idiosyncratic response to a vasoconstrictor such as a pseudoephedrine, or an overdose of such an OTC medication, may manifest itself as acute central nervous system stimulation. Added to the "adrenaline high" of performance in the actor or musical performer, the combination of effects may very well be deleterious. The patient who is unaware of these effects should be appraised of them promptly by the laryngologist.[2,34,36]

Phenobarbital and meprobamate are no longer commonly used as anxiolytics in the United States. Clomipramine (Anafranil) is useful in the anxiety evident in obsessive-compulsive disorder. The side effects are similar to tricyclic antidepressants: dry mouth, hypotension, constipation, tachycardia, sweating, tremor, and anorgasmia. Prozac has also proven effective for some patients with OCD and appears better tolerated.[34]

Hydroxyzine, an antihistamine, is occasionally prescribed for mild anxiety and/or pruritus. It does not produce physical dependence, but does potentiate the CNS effects of alcohol, narcotics, CNS depressants, and tricyclic antidepressants. Side effects include notable mucous membrane dryness and drowsiness. Buspirone (Buspar) is not sedating at its usual dosage levels and it has little addictive potential. Side effects include mild degrees of headache, nausea, and dizziness. However, it is poorly tolerated in patients accustomed to the more immediate relief of benzodiazepines.[34]

Various antipsychotic drugs have a mode of action that involves dopamine antagonism, probably in the mesolimbic or mesocortical areas.

They also have endocrine effects through dopamine receptors in the hypothalamic-pituitary axis.[34] The antipsychotic agents most commonly prescribed currently include haloperidol (Haldol, in various preparations), chlorpromazine hydrochloride (Thorazine), chlorpromazine hydrochloride (Sparine), fluphenazine hydrochloride (Prolixin), thioridazine (Mellaril), perphenazine (Trilafon), trifluoperazine hydrochloride (Stelazine), prochlorperazine (Compazine), molindone (Moban), loxapine hydrochloride (Loxitane), and clozapine (Clozaril). These potent agents have very significant side effects. Clozaril is used primarily in patients who are refractory to other neuroleptics and requires very close monitoring for bone marrow depression. Sedation, accompanied by fatigue during early dosing and akinesia with chronic administration, frequently are described. Anticholinergic effects include postural hypotension, dry mouth, nasal congestion, and constipation. The endocrine system is also affected, with a direct increase in blood prolactin levels. Breast enlargement and galactorrhea are seen in males and females and correlate with impotence and amenorrhea. Weight gain is often excessive and frequently leads to noncompliance. Skin complications such as rash, retinal pigmentation, and photosensitivity occur. Rare but serious complications include agranulocytosis, allergic obstructive hepatitis, seizures, and sudden death secondary to ventricular fibrillation.[34,36]

Approximately 14% of patients receiving long-term (greater than 7 years) treatment with antipsychotics agents will develop tardive dyskinesia ranging from minimal tongue restlessness to incapacitating, disfiguring choreiform and/or athetoid movements, especially of the head, neck, and hands. Unfortunately, there is no cure for the condition once it develops, nor are there accurate predictors for which patients will be affected.[34,36] One 1992 study suggested that therapy with vitamin E might moderate the symptoms of tardive dyskinesia.[40]

The mode of action producing neurologic side effects of the neuroleptics is primarily cholinergic-dopaminergic blockade. Dystonia usually involves tonic spasm of the tongue, jaw, and neck, but may range from mild tongue stiffness to opisthotonos.[34] Pseudo-parkinsonism may occur very early in treatment. Drug-induced parkinsonism occurs in 90% of cases within the first 72 days of treatment with a peak onset of 5–30 days.[9(p 29-135)] It is evidenced by muscle stiffness, cogwheel rigidity, stooped posture, masklike facies with loss of salivary control, dysarthria, and dysphagia. Pill-rolling tremor is rare. Akathisia, an inner-driven muscular restlessness with rhythmic leg jiggling, hand-wringing, and pacing, is extremely unpleasant. Multiple drug regimens are employed to diminish these symptoms.[34,36] A drug recently marketed which selectively blocks dopamine receptors without blocking receptors in the basal ganglia is risperidone (Risperdal).[39]

Neuroleptic malignant syndrome is a potentially fatal complication of these drugs. Patients will manifest hyperthermia, severe extra-pyramidal signs, and autonomic hyperarousal. Neuroleptics also affect temperature regulation generally and can predispose to heat stroke.[34,36]

Ongoing psychiatric treatment of patients with voice disorders mandates a careful evaluation of current and prior psychoactive drug therapy. In addition, numerous psychoactive substances are used in the medical management of neurological conditions such as Tourette's syndrome (haloperidol [Haldol], pimozide [Orac], and clonidine [Catapres]); chronic pain syndromes (carbamazepine, clonazepam); and vertigo (diazepam).

It is essential for laryngologists caring for professional singers to be familiar with these agents and alert for drug side effects and interactions. The numerous potential side effects of psychoactive medications highlight the importance of obtaining a good, comprehensive history. Some patients are reluctant to volunteer psychiatric information, especially to an ear, nose, and throat doctor when the relationship between psychiatric and voice treatment may not be obvious to the patient. It is critical to take the time to establish the rapport and patient confidence that permits acquisition of a complete, accurate history of psychological dysfunction and treatment. It is appropriate (with the patient's consent) to consult with the prescribing physician directly to advocate the use of the psychoactive drug least likely to produce adverse effects on the voice while adequately controlling the psychiatric illness.[2,9(p29-135)]

This chapter reviewed only a small number of the pharmacological agents that may have laryngeal side effects. Virtually all pharmaceutical and chemical agents may have adverse effects on the voice. It is essential for psychological professionals to be familiar with the vocal effects of any substance ingested by a voice patient and to warn all voice patients to discuss the potential vocal problems associated with even prescribed medication use with all of their physicians.

REFERENCES

1. Sataloff RT. *Professional Voice: The Science and Art of Clinical Care*, 2nd ed. San Diego, Calif: Singular Publishing Group Inc; 1997.
2. Sataloff RT, Lawrence VL, Hawkshaw MJ, Rosen DC. Medications and their effects on the voice. In: Benninger MS, Jacobson BH, Johnson AF, eds. *Vocal Arts Medicine: The Care and Prevention of Professional Voice Disorders*. New York, NY: Thieme Medical Publishers; 1994:216-225.

3. Davies WL, Gunert RR, Hoff RF, McGahen JW, et al. Antiviral activity of 1-Amantanamine (Amantadine). *Science*. 1964;144:862-863.
4. McGahen JW, Hoffmann CE. Influenza infections of mice. 1. Curative activity of Amantadine HCL. *Proc Soc Exp Biol Med*. 1968;129:678-681.
5. Wingfield WL, Pollock D, Gunert RR. Therapeutic efficacy of Amantadine-HCL and Rumantidine-HCL in naturally occurring influence A2 respiratory illness in man. *N Eng J Med*. 1969;281:579-584.
6. Council on Drugs. The Amantadine controversy. *JAMA*. 1967;201:372-373.
7. Feder RL. The professional voice and airline flight. *Otolaryngol Head Neck Surg*. 1984;92(3):251-254.
8. Sataloff RT. Professional singers: the science and art of clinical care. *Am J Otolaryngol*. 1981;2(3):251-266.
9. Vogel D, Carter J. *The Effects of Drugs on Communication Disorders*. San Diego, Calif: Singular Publishing Group Inc; 1995:47,29-135.
10. Punt NA. Applied laryngology—singers and actors. *Proc R Soc Med*. 1968;61:1152-1156.
11. Toogood JH, Jennings B, Greenway RW, Chuang L. Candidiasis and dysphonia complicating beclomethasone treatment of asthma. *J Allergy Clin Immunol*. 1980;65(2):145-153.
12. *Nursing '89 Drug Handbook*. Springhouse, Pa: Springhouse Corporation; 1989:236.
13. Martin FG. Drugs and vocal function. *J Voice*. 1988;2(4):338-344.
14. Lawrence VL. Medical care for professional voice (panel). In: Lawrence VL, ed. *Transcripts from the Annual Symposium: Care of the Professional Voice*. New York, NY: The Voice Foundation; 1978;3:17-18.
15. Schiff M. Medical management of acute laryngitis. In: Lawrence V, ed. *Transcripts of the Sixth Symposium: Care of the Professional Voice*. New York, NY: The Voice Foundation; 1977:99-102.
16. Damste PH. Virilization of the voice due to anabolic steroids. *Folia Phoniat*. 1964;16:10-18.
17. Damste PH. Voice changes in adult women caused by virilizing agents. *J Speech Hear Disord*. 1967;32:126-132.
18. Saez S, Francoise S. Recepteurs d'androgenes: mise en evidence dans la fraction cytosolique de muqueuse normale et d'epitheliomas pharyngolarynges humains. *CR Acad Sci* (Paris). 1975;280:935-938.
19. Vuorenkoski V, Lenko HL, Tjernlund P, Vuorenkoski L, Perheentupa J. Fundamental voice frequency during normal and abnormal growth, and after androgen treatment. *Arch Dis Child*. 1978;53:201-209.
20. Arndt HJ. Stimmstorungen nach Behandlung mit androgenen und anabolen Hormonen. *Munch Med Wochenschr*. 1974;116:1715-1720.
21. Bourdial J. Les troubles de la voix provoques par la therapeutique hormonale androgene. *Ann Otolaryngol* (Paris). 1970;87:725-734.
22. Dordain M. Étude statistique de l'influence des contraceptifs hormonaux sur la voix. *Folia Phoniat*. 1972;24:86-96.
23. Pahn V, Goretzlehner G. Stimmstorungen durch hormonale Kontrazeptiva. *Zentralb Gynakol*. 1978;100:341-346.

24. Schiff M. "The pill" in otolaryngology. *Trans Am Acad Ophthalmol Otolaryngol.* J-F 1968;72:76-84.
25. Brodnitz F. Medical care preventive therapy (panel). In: Lawrence V, ed. *Transcripts of the Seventh Annual Symposium: Care of the Professional Voice.* New York, NY: The Voice Foundation; 1978;3:86.
26. Carroll C. Arizona State University at Tempe: Unpublished research.
27. Bausch J. Wirkung und Nebenwirkung hormonaler Antikonzeptiva im Bereich von Nase, Hals und Ohr. *HNO.* 1983;31(12):409-414.
28. Können contraceptiva mit progestative Wirkung stemveranderingen verurzaken?. *Ned Tijdschr Geneeskd.* 1975;119(44):1726-1727.
29. Krahulec I, Urbanova O, Simko S. Prispevok kstudiu zmien hlasu pri hormonalnej antikoncepcii. *Cesk Otolaryngol.* 1977;26(4):234-237.
30. Wendler J. Zyklusabhangige Leistungsschwankungen der Stimme und ihre Beeinflussung durch Ovulationshemmer. *Folia Phoniatr* (Basel). 1972;24(4): 259-277.
31. James IM. The effects of oxprenolol on stage fright in musicians. *Lancet.* 1977;2:952-954.
32. Brantigan CD. The effect of beta blockage and beta stimulation on stage fright. *Am J Med.* 1982;72(1):88-94.
33. Gates GA, Saegert J, Wilson N, Johnson L, Sheperd A, Hearnd EM. Effects of beta-blockers on singing performance. *Ann Otol Rhinol Laryngol.* 1985:94:570-574.
34. Schatzberg A, Cole J. *Manual of Clinical Psychopharmacology,* 2nd ed. Washington, DC: APA Press; 1991:50, 110-125, 158-164, 169, 177, 185-227, 313-348.
35. Cole J, Bodkin J. Antidepressant drug side effects. *J Clin Psychiatry.* 1990;51(suppl 1):21-26.
36. Janitec P, Davis J, Prescorn F, Ab S. *Principles and Practice of Psychopharmacology.* Baltimore, Md: Williams and Wilkins; 1993:164-184, 230-289, 433-439.
37. Tornatore F, ed. *Psychopharmacology update.* Providence, RI: Manisses Communications Group Inc; 1996;7(2):7.
38. Wyeth Laboratories. Physician prescribing package information. Philadelphia, Pa: Wyeth Laboratories; 1983. Package insert for Effexor.
39. *Physicians' Desk Reference.* Oradell, NJ: Medical Economics Data; 1994;2000-2003, 2267-2270.
40. Egan M, Hyde T, Alvers A, Alexander M, Reeve A, Blom A, Saenz R, Wyatt R. Treatment of tardive dyskinesia with vitamin E. *Am J Psychiatr.* 1983;149(6):773-777.

CHAPTER

6

Psychological Assessment of Patients with Voice Disorders

Psychological care of voice professionals takes place within and as an adjunct to the medical treatment simultaneously being provided to these patients. The approaches described in this chapter reflect the theoretical and clinical techniques utilized by the author. When the psychological professional will be engaged in direct treatment of the patient, a formal diagnostic interview is conducted. When the clinician is offering consultation which will enhance the care provided by other voice team professionals (ie, laryngologist, speech-language pathologist, singing voice specialist, acting voice specialist, and nurse), information is gathered largely by assessment of verbal *content* gained during interviews conducted by other team members and by careful attention to the linguistic *processes* and parameters. These may include the use of sensory predicates (visual/auditory/kinesthetic/olfactory/gustatory), observation of the patient's habitual representational system, the use of personal metaphor, and nonverbal and paraverbal behaviors such as eye accessing patterns and the use of gesture. This information will allow the psychological professional to assist in increasing the effectiveness of interventions provided by others.

In individual psychotherapy, a confidential and intensive relationship develops between a patient with emotional and behavioral dysfunction and a skilled clinician who uses verbal and nonverbal methods to effect symptom relief and improve the patient's relationships with others and his or her ability to cope with internal and external stressors.[1] Care for voice professionals requires additional expertise in medical (health) psychology and arts medicine psychology. This type of counselling involves a more participative relationship between the patient who has a need to address health risks and/or change lifestyle patterns and a skilled, sensitized clinician who is aware of the inherent demands of performance.[2] This expertise allows the clinician to more empathically "join" the world of the performer and to be considered competent and credible by him or her. A high level of accurate empathy can facilitate the patient's acquisition and maintenance of beneficial psychological and physiological changes.

The duration of treatment is usually short-term. Methods are action-oriented and involve information giving and suggestions for more adaptive lifestyle behaviors, as well as a number of traditional psychotherapeutic interventions. Whenever possible, the therapist should have reviewed the medical record of the patient and become familiar with all available information. This information should offer the therapist hypotheses with regard to the emotional issues that may be present. Of course, the first task of the therapist in any initial interview is to create a climate in which the patient can begin to relax and focus on what he or she needs and wants, establishing a relationship that can make helping possible. Within this context, the task is to gather enough information from the patient to make preliminary decisions about what to do, whether to offer therapy, and what the therapeutic goals will be. The focus of the interview is to contact the individual's emotional pain and create an alliance with the patient that permits identifying the problems that are hidden by habitual defenses.[3(p36-50),4(p 33-38)]

During the entire evaluation, the therapist not only interacts with the patient, but also simultaneously observes the interaction carefully and critically. Psychological evaluation requires the examiner to perform the challenging task of grasping in a limited amount of time the past and present difficulties that prompt the patient to consult a mental health professional. The goal is to discover the nature and intensity of the patient's inner conflicts, the extent to which they interfere with important areas of functioning, and whether they warrant therapeutic intervention. If so, the evaluation should lead to selection of the most appropriate approach. These patients have presented themselves for medical assessment and treatment of their voice-related concerns. Psychological assessment may have come only as a result of referrals made by the laryngologist or other members of the treatment team. Patients' degree of investment in adjunctive psychological care may, therefore, vary widely. A critical question to be answered in the very early phases is, "What led you to seek help from me at this particular time?"

At the beginning of the initial interview, it does not really matter where the client starts; what matters is that he or she begins to experience the quality of the relationship which will be built throughout the course of treatment. Rapport has several components, including putting the patient and the therapist at ease, finding the pain and expressing compassion, evaluating the patient's insight and becoming an ally, demonstrating expertise, establishing authority as a therapist, and balancing the roles in the therapeutic setting.[5]

The therapist must find a way to allow the patient to tell his or her story. Some parts obviously are especially important, and other parts will require later clarification. Initially, the patient should be encouraged to follow his or her own agenda, to talk about whatever is in the "foreground." The author (DCR) prefers to begin with an opening statement such as "I'd like to know something about you and how you decided to come for therapy at this time. Where would you like to begin? Later on, I will probably have specific questions; but for right now, I'd like you to talk about whatever you most want to tell me today."

As the conversation progresses, the therapist listens at many levels. The most obvious level is that of content, and the patient has a right to expect that the therapist will remember and understand remarks in the context of what has previously been said. Nonverbal communication is critical: this includes posture, voice tone, facial expression, eye accessing patterns, the use of gesture, pauses, and silence. The nonverbal and paraverbal communications of the patient provide constant commentary and the opportunity to assess for congruence with the actual words. Another level of listening is that of style: the pattern and rhythm of the dialogue, its coherence and logic, and the patient's active versus passive stance. Morsund states that "the therapy hour is a microcosm of the patient's whole pattern of interacting with the world, and much can be learned about his/her social relationships, sense of self, strengths, and weakness by attending to the overall ebb and flow of the first therapy interaction."[3(p41)]

A formal diagnostic psychiatric assessment will be reported. So, whether the therapist is most comfortable using systematic questioning or a more patient-directed narrative, the information must nevertheless be reported in a meaningful and organized form. We prefer a traditional format. The record will begin with identifying data including demographic information and the referring source. The chief complaint is reported verbatim. The history of the present illness is formatted in an orderly chronological fashion by the psychological professional and will include the nature and intensity of the patient's conflicts, previous episodes of psychological symptomatology, previous treatment and outcomes; and the patient's level of insight with regard to the presenting symptoms. The record should include a summary of the patient's personal history with emphasis on events in the past not covered in the preceding category. This will include predictable crises in the individual's development from infancy, including childhood, adolescence, and adulthood. Reference should be made to the patient's educational and occupational history, social history, sexual and relationship history, family history, and medical history, including prior and current drug therapy.

The purpose of the mental status examination is to observe and record in a systematic way the current emotional state and specific mental functions of the patient. The categories used are intended primarily to help organize and record data. The therapist explores most of these features while taking the psychological history. The following features are assessed: general appearance, attitude toward the psychological symptoms and toward the therapist, motor behavior, pitch and rate of speech, affective states and the patient's subjective description of mood, thought processes, thought content, clarity of perception, level of intellectual functioning, orientation to time, place, and person, memory for recent and past events, judgment, and personal and social resources.[6,7] (See Appendix I.)

Psychological diagnosis is an extremely protracted process, and the therapeutic process becomes, paradoxically, a "diagnostic intervention in which the inner situation of the patient unfolds in an ever sharpening form . . . equally paradoxically, the diagnostic process is in itself the therapeutic process."[7(p132)] It is often impossible to make an accurate diagnosis on the basis of one assessment session, especially with an anxious, distraught, defensive, or ambivalent patient. However, for the purposes of third-party payment, it is often necessary to generate a diagnosis using the DSM-IV criteria. The therapist would do well to remember that any psychological diagnosis is an abstraction, a set of categories that may or may not provide a good fit for what the patient is reporting and demonstrating. Diagnosis is at best an approximation for what is true for any individual, and it is subject to change as more is learned about the patient. Morsund counsels that there is a great temptation after having made a diagnosis to use it to filter all subsequent information and to create a self-fulfilling prophecy. She reiterates the concern that initial diagnoses tend to take on a life of their own; "like weeds in the garden, they tend to persist beyond the time when we believe we have chopped them down and replaced them with something more useful."[2(p44)] Hence, it is reasonable to put forth a working diagnosis that will assist the patient toward receiving needed therapy, as long as the therapist remains comfortable with the fluidity of diagnostic labels during the therapeutic process.

The reasons for diagnostic psychological interviewing in this setting are many. They include a search for history of prior psychopathology or co-morbid psychologic illness, response to prior life or health crises, an understanding of the patient's intra- and interpersonal resources for support, the ethical issues related to interaction with psychological colleagues currently providing care to the patient, and the need for the development and documentation of a treatment plan. Providing holistic care to performers requires attention to all the domains of their existence. Indeed, failure to address the psychological and social concomitants of medical illness in this population often leads to attenuation or failure of the medical treatment regimen and suboptimal surgical outcome.

The psychological professional serving as a member of the voice team will expand the traditional psychological assessment to focus on several areas of specific interest. One of these includes a functional assessment, that is, "How does your voice problem interfere with your daily life?" This question is followed by an inquiry about the life tasks of work, love, family, and friendship, including the individual's level of functioning and degree of satisfaction with each of these tasks. The extent of distress and impairment often is related to receptivity to change. The more distressed the individual, the more responsive he or she may be to a treatment program that will relieve that distress and impairment.

A second question involves the patient's unique and personal explanation for the current symptom or condition, in symbolic terms, the importance of the event to the individual. In a psychological sense, it is the emotional meaning that the symptom has for the individual that is all-important and predicts the type of reaction that will follow impairment or loss. The patient is asked, "What do you believe is the reason for this voice problem?" The answer to this and follow-up questions begins to suggest the patient's individual health beliefs, attributions, and the extent of the factual accuracy regarding the diagnosis and prognosis.

A third question helps to elicit the patient's expectations for treatment in terms of involvement of time and effort, expected outcome, and measures of satisfaction. The inquiry, "What specific changes are you expecting as a result of our work together? How will we both be able to know when these have occurred?" is posed. The therapist should evaluate all of the patient's previous attempts to address the psychological symptoms. An attempt at helping the patient report his or her earliest recollection of experiences of significant illness may be helpful in assessing the customary stance toward the patient role. Often, these responses provide valuable insights into a person's body image and cognitions or beliefs about self and other people. The silent attitudes and norms of the patient's family, social and ethnic group, and community influence and reinforce certain health beliefs and not others.[3(p10-17),8]

Psychological assessment needs to be tailored to the special characteristics of the population for whom the therapist provides care. Arts medicine psychologists work with injured or potentially injured performers. Specialized assessment techniques have been developed to address the issues common to disability. All humans are subjected to losses and separations throughout their lives. So, why is it that some people cope maladaptively, and why only after some events? An individual manifests stress responses which arise from a particular set of circumstances in the life setting. This engenders an emotional cascade that depends on the specific meaning the experience of loss has to that person. The degree of individual stress of an event is highly distinctive; stress arising from a particular diagnosis is a function of the way it is perceived by that individual, rather than a function of the diagnosis itself.[9] The perception of injury is only a potential stress. What makes it an actual stressor is the impact it has on the affected individual.

Carl Rogers suggested that one motivational tendency of human beings is to make self-concept congruent with life experience. The most common definition of self-concept is those feelings, evaluations, and perceptions of oneself that define who one is. Rogers' elaboration of the self-concept, and his conceptualization of the "real self" versus "ideal self" discrepancy, have contributed significantly to our understanding of the impact of any disability on the individual. Because individuals' self-concept, values, feelings, and judgments of self guide their behavior, it follows that it is not disability per se that psychologically influences the person, but rather the subjective meanings and feelings attached to the disability. The "real self" versus "ideal self" discrepancy becomes critical when patients view themselves differently as a result of a voice disorder from the way they wish to view themselves.[10]

A premise of the authors' work is that professional voice users with significant lasting changes in vocal quality or stamina experience a serious threat to self-definition and self-image. When the change is permanent, they must acknowledge and grieve the loss of a body part and release the associated negative emotions. When the prognosis is uncertain, vocal professionals will move through several phases of emotional adjustment which necessitate reality testing and appropriately tailored psychological interventions. Of special interest during assessment are current and cumulative psychological stressors, especially loss and significant changes in lifestyle. The pattern of coping responses must be assessed for its ability to aid in positive adaptation to a diagnosis of voice impairment.

In addition to the diagnostic interview previously described, patients receiving psychological care at the voice center complete a number of paper and pencil questionnaires. This is done at the beginning of treatment for purposes of research and ongoing calibration of their responses to therapy, as well as at two other specified points during the psychotherapeutic treatment. (See Appendix I.) The first instrument asks for self-report data with regard to demographics and the patient's description of his or her voice use and voice problem, as well as a rough chronology of prior treatment. The second is modification of the Holmes and Rahe scale.[11] The third asks patients to evaluate their stress management strategies. This information is used in designing a personalized stress management repertoire. Next, patients are asked to describe their loss histories using an open question format, and to indicate any and all reactions they experience in the categories of affect, physical sensations, behaviors, and cognitions. This is a form modified from the work of Worden.[12]

Finally, projective art is used. Rather than being evaluated as psychometric instruments, these art techniques are regarded by the authors as clinical tools and serve as supplementary, qualitative interviewing aids. At three different times throughout treatment, the patient is given two 8½ × 11 inch sheets of white paper. A fresh box of 64 crayons is provided, and the patient is instructed to, "Draw yourself." On the second sheet, the instruction is, "Draw your voice." The theoretical premise is that the individual not only reveals his or her emotional struggles, but may experience some catharsis in doing so and discussing the experience underlies this request. These two modifications of the Draw-a-Person test will be described in more detail in Chapters 10 and 17.[11,13]

This has been a most fruitful form of assessment with these artist-patients. It is perhaps paradoxical intervention: by prohibiting their most familiar and highly developed form of artistry (and thereby relieving the attendant performance anxiety) but providing another artistic outlet, their inner worlds could be "given voice" visually. Miller has expressed this dilemma of the psychological sciences:

> In its understandable effort to be regarded as one of the natural sciences, psychology paid the unnecessarily high price of setting aside any consideration of consciousness and purpose, in the belief that such concepts would plunge the discipline back into a swamp of metaphysical idealism. Research was designed on "positivistic" lines so that emphasis inevitably fell on measurable stimuli and observable behavior. It soon became apparent that such a direction could not be long sustained and that psychology would begin to stagnate if research failed to take account the inner state of the living being.[14(p32)]

According to Jung, the "inner state" finds its entrance into consciousness through art.[15] Carolyn Kenny's work on music therapy describes this inner experience as the creation of a new language with which to grasp more fully the processes leading toward human change, and its practitioners as those who "see the vision and hear the song of the one and the many, those who can guard the threshold of being and who wait for sound."[16(p xiv-xv)]

This is the rightful role of the arts medicine psychologist: to possess mastery of the knowledge bases of psychology and medicine and also an experiential understanding of the performing arts so that he or she may stand in alliance with the injured performer on the journey to explore, understand, and modify the psychological impact of performance-related injuries.

REFERENCES

1. Singer E. *Key Concepts in Psychotherapy*. New York, NY: Random House; 1965:132.
2. Sperry L, Carlson J, Lewis J. Health counselling strategies and interventions. *J Ment Health Counselling*. 1993;15:15-25.
3. Moursund J. *The Process of Counselling and Therapy*. Englewood Cliffs, NJ: Prentice-Hall Inc; 1985:36-50.
4 Hislop I. Stress, *Distress, and Illness*. Sydney: McGraw-Hill Book Co; 1991:33-38.
5. Othmer E, Othmer S. *The Clinical Interview Using DSM-III-R*. Washington, DC: American Psychiatric Press Inc; 1989:16.
6. Nicholi A, ed. *The New Harvard Guide to Psychiatry*. Cambridge, MA: The Belknap Press of Harvard University Press; 1988:29-45.
7. Waldinger R. *Psychiatry for Medical Students*. Washington, DC: American Psychiatric Press Inc; 1984:3-77.
8. Sperry L, Carlson J, Lewis J. Health counselling strategies and interventions. *J Mental Health Counselling*. 1993;15:15-25.
9. Lazarus RS. The concepts of stress and disease. In: Levy L, ed. *Society, Stress, and Disease*. London: Oxford University Press; 1971:53-58.
10. Parker R, Hanson C. *Rehabilitation Counselling*. Boston, MA: Allyn and Bacon Inc; 1981:147-149.
11. Anastasi A. *Psychological Testing*, 6th ed. New York, NY: Macmillan Publishing Co; 1988:599-622.
12. Worden JW. Grief *Counseling and Grief Therapy: A Handbook for the Mental Health Practitioner*. New York, NY: Springer Publishing Company; 1982:7-34.
13. Furth G. *The Secret World of Drawings: Healing Through Art*. Boston, MA: Sigo Press; 1988:18-34.
14. Miller J. *States of Mind*. New York, NY: Pantheon Books; 1983:32.

15. Jung CC. *Symbols of Transformation*. Princeton, NJ: Princeton University Press; 1956:5.
16. Kenny C. *The Field of Play: A Guide for the Theory and Practice of Music Therapy*. Atascadero, CA: Ridgeview Publishing Co; 1989:xiv-xv.

CHAPTER

7

Co-Morbid Psychopathology

The psychological professional functioning as a member of a voice care treatment team, or as a community clinician to whom referrals of voice patients are made, will be familiar with the broad range of psychiatric illness. This chapter provides only the briefest of reviews of major psychopathology and its presentations. The only material unfamiliar to psychological professionals may be the voice and speech manifestations common to various psychiatric syndromes. The summary also may be useful when psychological professionals function in the role of educator to colleagues and peers, including the referring otolaryngologist, speech-language pathologist, or singing teacher.

As physicians, otolaryngologists receive some training in general psychiatry as medical students. However, unless they are particularly psychologically minded, their theoretical and clinical experience rarely goes beyond that point. The registered nurse serving on a voice treatment team frequently is the first professional to assess the psychosocial adjustment of the patient. He or she is educated to be particularly sensitive to holistic care. Speech-language pathologists receive varying degrees of emphasis on counseling in their graduate programs. Stemple states that voice pathologists must develop superior interview skills, counseling skills, and the skill to know when emotional or psychosocial elements require more intensive evaluation and therapy by other professionals.[1] Andrews, who has a particular interest in the psychological aspects of voice disorders, believes that speech-language pathologists should take a greater counseling role in the treatment of the voice-injured patient. "Mental health counselors can help patients understand the psychosocial dynamics of voice problems, but only speech-language pathologists can help patients produce and habituate more appropriate vocal behaviors. The speech-language pathologist's ability to help patients integrate new insights about their feelings and relationships into their communication strategies is significant."[2(p384)] She cautions that the major thrust of the psychosocial aspects of treatment by speech-language pathologists should be to identify and understand the factors that impinge on vocal behavior.[2] Singing voice teachers receive little or no education in their pedagogy courses about the impact of emotion and its conveyance on voice. Although they serve by default as counselors to their students, formal counseling skills and the recognition of psychopathology are not within their scope of practice. The psychological professional's role includes significant peer education.

Otolaryngologists and all other health care providers involved with patients with voice disorders should recognize significant co-morbid psychopathology. Patterns of voice use may provide clues to the presence of psychopathology, although voice disturbance is certainly not the principal feature of major psychiatric illness. Nevertheless, failure to recognize serious psychopathology in voice patients may result not only in errors in voice diagnosis and failures of therapy, but more importantly in serious injury to the patient, sometimes even death.

Although a full depressive syndrome, including melancholia, can occur as a result of loss, it fulfills the criteria for a major depressive episode when the individual becomes preoccupied with feelings of worthlessness and guilt, demonstrates marked psychomotor retardation, and becomes impaired in both social and occupational function.[3] Careful listening during the taking of a history will reveal flat affect including slowed rate of speech, decreased length of utterance, lengthy pauses, decreased pitch variability, monoloudness, and frequent use of vocal fry.[4,5] William Styron described his speech during his depressive illness as "slowed to the vocal equivalent of a shuffle."[6]

Major depression may be part of the patient's past medical history, may be a "co-morbid illness," or may be a result of the presenting problem. The essential feature is a prominent, persistent dysphoric mood characterized by a loss of pleasure in nearly all activities. Appetite and sleep are disturbed, and there may be marked weight gain or loss, hypersomnia, or one of three insomnia patterns. Psychomotor agitation or retardation may be present. Patients may demonstrate distractibility, memory disturbances, and difficulty concentrating. Feelings of worthlessness, helplessness, and hopelessness are a classic triad. Suicidal ideation, with or without plan, and/or concomitant psychotic features may necessitate emergency intervention.

Major affect disorders are classified as unipolar or bipolar. In bipolar disorder, the patient will also experience periods of mania, a recurrent elated state first occurring in young adulthood. (First manic episodes in patients over 50 should alert the clinician for medical or central nervous system [CNS] illness or to the effects of drugs.) The presentation of the illness includes the following major characteristics on a continuum of severity: elevated mood, irritability/hostility, distractibility, inflated self-concept, grandiosity, physical and sexual overactivity, flight of ideas, decreased need for sleep, social intrusiveness, buying sprees, and inappropriate collections of possessions. Manic patients demonstrate impaired social and familial behavior patterns. They are manipulative, alienate family members, and tend to have a very high divorce rate.[3,7] Vocal presentation will manifest flight of ideas (content), rapid paced, pressured speech, and often increased pitch and volume. There may be dysfluency related to the rate of speech, breathlessness, and difficulty in interrupting the language stream. Three major theories based on neuroanatomy, neuroendocrinology, and neuropharmacology are the most currently promulgated explanations for these disease states, but they are beyond the scope of this chapter.[8,9]

Treatment of affective disorders includes psychotherapy. Diagnosis and short-term treatment of reactive depressive states may be performed by the psychologist on the voice team utilizing individual or group therapy modalities. Longer term treatment necessitates a referral to a community-based psychotherapist, ideally one whose skills, training, and understanding of the medical and artistic components of the illness are well known to the referring laryngologist, speech-language pathologist, or singing teacher. The use of psychopharmacologic agents is a risk/benefit decision. When the patient's symptom severity meets the criteria for major affective disorder, the physiologic effects of the disease, as well as the potential for self-destructive behavior, must be carefully considered.

Anxiety is an expected response in reaction to any medical diagnosis and the required treatment. Vocal presentations of anxiety vary with the continuum of psychiatric symptoms ranging from depression to agitation and including impairment of concentration. Psychotherapy, including desensitization, cognitive/behavioral techniques, stress management, hypnosis, and insight-oriented approaches, is helpful. Patients must learn to tolerate their distress factors and identify factors that precipitate or intensify their symptoms (see Chapter 15). Medication may be used to treat underlying depression and decrease the frequency of episodes. However, it leaves the underlying conflict unresolved and negatively affects artistic quality.[10,11] Some medical conditions are commonly associated with the presenting symptom of anxiety. These include CNS disease, Cushing's syndrome, hyperthyroidism, hypoglycemia, the consequences of minor head trauma, premenstrual syndrome, and cardiac disease such as mitral valve prolapse and various arrhythmias. Medications prescribed for other conditions may have anxiety as a side effect. These include such drugs as amphetamines, corticosteroids, caffeine, decongestants, cocaine, and the asthma armamentarium.[9]

Although psychotic behavior may be observed with major affective disorders, organic CNS disease, or drug toxicity, schizophrenia occurs in only 1%–2% of the general population.[12] Its onset is most prominent in mid- to late adolescence through the late 20s. Incidence is approximately equal for males and females, and schizophrenia has been described in all cultures and socioeconomic classes. This is a group of mental disorders that includes massive disruptions in cognition or perception, such as delusions, hallucinations, or thought disorders. The fundamental causes of schizophrenia are unknown, but the disease involves excessive amounts of neurotransmitters, chiefly dopamine. Genetic predisposition is present. Somatic delusions may present as voice complaints. However, flattening or inappropriateness of affect, a diagnostic characteristic of schizophrenia, will produce voice changes similar to those described for depression and mania. Where hallucinatory material creates fear, characteristics of anxiety and agitation will be audible. Perseveration, repetition, and neologisms may be present. The signs and symptoms also include clear indications of deterioration in social and occupational functioning, personal hygiene, changes in behavior and movement, an altered sense of self, and the presence of blunted or inappropriate affect.[3,5,13] The disease is chronic, and control requires consistent use of antipsychotic medications for symptom management. Social support in regulating activities of daily living is crucial in maintaining emotional control. Family counseling and support groups offer the opportunity to share experiences and resources in the care of this difficult disease.

EATING DISORDERS AND SUBSTANCE ABUSE

Rapport with the laryngologist and other voice team members also may allow patients to reveal other self-defeating disorders. The psychologist will inquire about these directly if a formal psychological evaluation is scheduled. Among the most common in arts medicine are body dysmorphic (eating) disorders and substance abuse problems. Comprehensive discussion of these subjects is beyond the scope of this chapter, but it is important for the treating professionals to recognize these conditions not only because of their effects on voice, but also because of the potentially serious general medical and psychiatric implications. In addition to posterior laryngitis and pharyngitis, laryngeal findings associated with bulimia include subepithelial vocal fold hemorrhages, superficial telangiectasia of the vocal fold mucosa, and vocal fold scarring.[14] Bulimia is a disorder associated with self-induced vomiting following episodes of binge eating. It may occur sporadically, or it may be a chronic problem. Vomiting produces signs and symptoms similar to severe chronic reflux, as well as thinning of tooth enamel. Bulimia nervosa can be a serious disorder and may be associated with anorexia nervosa. Bulimia may be more common than is commonly realized. It has been estimated to occur in as many as 2%–4% of female adolescents and female young adults.[15] Laryngologists must be attentive to the potential for anorexia and exercise addiction in the maintenance of a desirable body appearance in professional performers.

Alcohol, benzodiazepines, stimulants, cocaine, and narcotics are notoriously readily available in the performing community and "on the streets." Patients who demonstrate signs and symptoms, or who admit that these areas of their lives are out of control, have taken the first step to regaining control; and this should be acknowledged while efficiently arranging treatment. The window of opportunity often is remarkably narrow. The physician should establish close ties to excellent treatment facilities where specialized clinicians can offer confidential outpatient management, with inpatient care available when required for safety.

The psychological professional will recognize the extremely superficial treatment of the important diagnoses in this chapter. It is intended to be a ready reference and an accessible teaching tool for psychoeducation of patients or colleagues. The reader is referred to standard texts for a more thorough treatment of each subject[7,15,17] and to the DSM-IV for diagnostic and coding information.[3]

REFERENCES

1. Stemple JC, Glaze LE, Gerdeman BK. *Clinical Voice Pathology: Theory and Management,* 2nd ed. San Diego, Calif: Singular Publishing Group Inc; 1995:169.
2. Andrews ML. *Manual of Voice Treatment: Pediatrics Through Geriatrics* (Clinical Competence Series). San Diego, Calif: Singular Publishing Group Inc; 1995:384-385.
3. American Psychiatric Association. *Diagnostic and Statistical Manual of Mental Disorder III-R.* American Psychiatric Association: Washington DC; 1987:206-210.
4. Rosen DC, Sataloff RT. Psychological aspects of voice disorders. In: Rubin JS, Sataloff RT, Korovin GS, Gould WJ, eds. *Diagnosis and Treatment of Voice Disorders.* New York, NY: Igaku Shoin Medical Publishers; 1995:491-501.

5. Vogel D, Carter J. *The Effects of Drugs on Communication Disorders*. San Diego, CA: Singular Publishing Group Inc; 1995:31-143.
6. Styron N. *Darkness Visible: A Memoir of Madness*. New York, NY: Random House; 1990.
7. Klerman G. Depression and related disorders of mood. In: Nicholi A, ed. *The New Harvard Guide to Psychiatry*. Cambridge, MA: Harvard University Press; 1988:309-336.
8. Weissman M. The psychological treatment of depression: evidence for the efficacy of psychotherapy alone, in comparison with and in combination with pharmacotherapy. *Arch Gen Psychiatry*. 1979;38:1261-1269.
9. Ross E, Rush A. Diagnosis and neuroanatomical correlates of depression in brain-damaged patients: implications for a neurology of depression. *Arch Gen Psychiatry*. 1981;38:1344-1354.
10. Osterwald P, Avery M. Psychiatric problems of performing artists. In: Sataloff RT, Brandfonbrenner A, Lederman R, eds. *Textbook of Performing Arts Medicine*. New York, NY: Raven Press; 1991:319-335.
11. Sataloff RT. Stress, anxiety and psychogenic dysphonia. In: Sataloff RT, *Professional Voice: The Science and Art of Clinical Care*. New York, NY: Raven Press; 1991:195-200.
12. Tsuang M, Faraone S, Day M. Schizophrenic disorders. In: Nicholi A, ed. *The New Harvard Guide to Psychiatry*. Cambridge, MA: Harvard University Press; 1988:259-295.
13. *Physicians Desk Reference*. Oradell, NJ: Medical Economics Data; 1994:2000-2003, 2267-2270.
14. Sataloff RT. *Professional Voice: The Science and Art of Clinical Care*. New York, NY: Raven Press; 1991.
15. Kaplan H, Sadock B, eds. *Comprehensive Textbook of Psychiatry*, 4th ed. Baltimore, Md: Williams and Wilkins; 1985.
16. Maneros A, Tsuang M, eds. *Schizo-Affective Psychoses*. Berlin: Springer-Verlag; 1986.
17. Rush A, ed. *Short-Term Psychotherapies for Depression*. New York, NY: Guilford Press; 1982.

CHAPTER

8

Voice Professionals: Special Psychological Considerations

I t is useful to understand in greater depth the problems experienced by professional voice users who suffer vocal injuries. Most of the authors' observations of this population occurred among singers and actors. Although they are the most obvious and demanding professional voice users, many other professionals are classified as professional voice users, as noted in Chapter 3. Clinicians expect profound emotional reactions to voice problems among singers and actors, but many other patients demonstrate similar reactions. If these reactions are not recognized, they may be misinterpreted as anger, malingering, or other "difficult patient" behavior. Some patients are unconsciously afraid that their voices are "lost forever" and are psychologically unable to make a full effort at vocal recovery following injury or surgery. This blocking of the frightening possibilities by rationalization ("I haven't made a maximum attempt so I don't know yet if my voice will be satisfactory") can result in prolonged or incomplete recovery following technically flawless surgery. It is incumbent on the members of the voice team to understand the psychological consequences of voice disturbance and to recognize them not only in extreme cases, but even in their more subtle manifestations.

Typical successful professional voice users (especially actors, singers, and politicians) may fall into a personality subtype which is ambitious, driven, perfectionistic, and tightly controlled. Externally, they present themselves as confident, competitive, and self-assured. Internally, self-esteem, the product of personality development, often is far more fragile. Children and adolescents do the best they can to survive and integrate their life experience. All psychological defense mechanisms are means to that end. Most of these defenses are not under conscious control. They are a habitual element of the fabric of one's response to life, especially in stressful or psychologically threatening situations.

It is the task of personality theorists to explain this process, the genesis of the "self." There are numerous coherent personality theories, all substantially interrelated. The framework of Karen Horney (1885–1952) is particularly useful in attempting to understand the creative personality and its vulnerabilities.[1] In simplification, she formulated a "holistic notion of the personality as an individual unit functioning within a social framework and continually interacting with its environment."[(p185-186)] In Horney's model, there are three "selves." The *actual self* is the sumtotal of the individual's experience; the *real self* is responsible for harmonious integration; and the *idealized self* has set up unrealistically high expectations which, in the face of disappointment, result in self-hatred and self-alienation.[1] Horney's theory is used by the authors as a working model in evolving therapeutic approaches to this special patient population. They are the laryngologist's most demanding "consumers of voice care and cling to their physicians' explanations with dependency."[2(p523)]

All psychological adjustment expresses itself through the personality of the patient, and it is essential to focus on the personality style of every performer who seeks psychological help. This can best be done during psychological assessment and evaluation by exploring daily activities, especially those pertaining to the performer's involvement with his or her art, the patient's growth and personality development as an artist, and relationships with people both within and outside his or her performing environment. Each developmental phase carries inherent coping tasks and responsibilities which can play an important part in the patient's emotional response to vocal dysfunction. Musical training usually begins during childhood, a critical early phase of psychological development. Ostwald observes that the artistic child is, by virtue of his or her emerging talent, "different" from peers and family and therefore vulnerable.[3] Pruett argues that this vulnerability is not necessarily a risk unless it interacts with negative environmental factors such as unsupportive parental or educator attitudes toward the talented child.[4] Both Ostwald and Pruett[3,4] highlight adolescence as a period of risk not only for its rapid physical growth, sexual maturation, and identity formulation, but for the influence of peer relationships. They discuss the potential for crisis: a dangerous opportunity. The talented musical performer must determine whether his or her gift is owned by him or by significant others in his or her life. Competitiveness is a major factor in personality development as well. The process of musical development tends to encourage competition, as does the jury system in music conservatories. Ostwald notes that competitiveness is a factor in strengthening technical perfection, but the cost may be the artistry itself. The unhealthy atmosphere of overwork may produce a one-sided, constricted personality throughout adult life.[3]

The life tasks of adulthood require consolidation of personality and the making of life commitments which will have lasting effects on a performer's career. Decisions regarding a partner and possible parenthood pose logistical challenges for performers who must travel in order to pursue artistic opportunities, and struggles ensue between the psychobiological needs for intimacy, privacy, and family life and performance opportunities. Aging brings about changes in physical and cognitive abilities in all human beings, albeit at different rates. The performer faces loss of accustomed patterns of activity and his or her individual perceptions of growing old. Additionally, competition from younger performers may be ever present.[3]

The gift of great vocal talent carries a cost. To those to whom much is given, much is indeed expected. The developmental tasks of a performer carry with them special risks. For example, midlife reflections revolve around not only personal and social accomplishments, but also unfulfilled goals and career disappointments. Ostwald notes that professional burn-out may become a problem for the performer just as it does for other highly successful individuals. Some patients may cope with this by developing new life interests; others may experience dysphoria which may progress to depression.[3] For extremely successful performers there is danger of competition from younger artists along with the first signs of loss of vocal prowess. Not to be performing, no matter what the reason, is one of the most serious emotional risks for artists who have been in the spotlight since childhood. Their self-esteem depends heavily on public acclaim and continual audience reinforcement.[3,5] Pruett notes that, regardless of our professional discipline, "we all lose our performing careers one way or another."[4(p348)] Learning about, cherishing, and learning to manage our unique, individual psychological vulnerabilities is critical to adaptive psychological function throughout life.

Research into body image theory also provides a theoretical basis for understanding the special impact of threats or injuries to the voice in vocal performers. The body is essential to all perception, learning, and memory; and the body serves as a sensory register and processor of sensory information. Body experience is deeply personal and constitutes a private world typically shared with others only under conditions of closest intimacy. Moreover, the body is an expressive instrument, the medium through which individuality is communicated verbally and nonverbally.[6] It is therefore possible to anticipate direct correspondence between certain physical illness or injury and body and self-image. Among these are psychosomatic conditions and/or body states with high levels of involvement of personality factors. In these cases, body illness or injury may reactivate psychopathological processes that began in early childhood or induce an emotional disorder such as denial or inappropriately prolonged depression.[6] Psychological reactions to a physical injury are not uniformly disturbing or distressing and do not necessarily result in maladjustment. However, Shontz[6] notes that reactions to body injury are more a function of how much anxiety is generated by the experience than by the actual location, severity, or type of injury itself.

Patients are notoriously adaptive and capable of living with most types of difficulties, injuries, or disabilities if they feel there is a good reason for doing so. If one's life has broad meaning and purpose, any given disorder takes on less significance. When a physical disability or any given body part becomes the main focus of concern or has been the main source of self-esteem in a person's life, that life becomes narrowed and restricted. Patients adapt satisfactorily to a personal medical condition when the problems of living related to the injury cease to be the dominant element in their total psychological life.

A unique closeness exists between one's body and one's identity; this body-self is a central part of self-concept. The interdependence of body image and self-esteem means that distortion of one will affect the other. The cognitive-behavioral model for understanding body image includes perceptual and affective components, as well as attitudinal ones. From the cognitive perspective, any body image producing dysphoria results from irrational thoughts, unrealistic expectations, and faulty explanations.[7] Body image constructs and their affective and cognitive outcomes relate to personality types and cognitive styles. For example, depressive personality types chronically interpret events in terms of deficiencies and are trapped by habitual self-defeating thoughts. Anxious personality types chronically overestimate risks and become hypervigilant. These types of cognitive errors generate automatic thoughts which intensify body image-related psychopathology.

The psychological professional providing care to this special population must be well versed in developmental psychology, experience the world of the performer, and retain an unshakable empathy for the extraordinary psychologically disorganizing impact of potential vocal injury. It is critical to harken back to one of the earliest lessons taught to all psychotherapists-in-training. That is, the therapist must, through accurate empathy, earn the right to make interpretations and interventions. When this type of insightful and accurate support is available to the professional voice user, the psychotherapist may well be the patient's rudder in the rough seas of diagnosis, treatment, and rehabilitation.

Punt has described the personalities of professional actors and singers as intense, volatile, excitable, emotional, neurotic, anxious, temperamental, moody, intemperate, vain, and unstable.[8] He further taught that, in times of extreme stress, even the trained voice user will project emotional problems into the voice, affecting voice quality and its precision of movement. Although Punt's reflections on the personality attributes of performers may be questionable, any person's emotional or mental state can have an effect on vocal production. "Non-artistic" professional voice users also demonstrate personality factors that put their voices at risk. Salespersons are most successful when they are focused and intense in their communication patterns. Clergy are subjected to enormous emotional demands as they minister to the personal needs and distress of their congregants. Educators may be anxious about the responsibility of educating their students and the evaluations which permit them to compete for promotions and tenure. Prominent lecturers in all disciplines rely on the strength of their content material, but also on the polish of their presentation, to retain their professional celebrity and financial success. Personality characteristics which are inherent in professional voice users, along with the impact of exogenous and endogenous stress, may all contribute to voice use patterns that may result in voice disorders.[8]

REFERENCES

1. Meissner W. Theories of personality. In: Nicholi A, ed. *The New Harvard Guide to Psychiatry*. Cambridge, Mass: Harvard University Press; 1988:177-199.
2. Ray CJ, Fitzgibbon G. Socially mediated reduction of stress in surgical patients. In: Oborne DJ, Grunberg M, Eisner JR, eds. *Research and Psychology in Medicine*. Oxford: Pergamon Press; 1979;2:521-527.
3. Ostwald P, Avery M. Psychiatric problems of performing artists. In: Sataloff RT, Brandfonbrener A, Lederman R, eds. *Textbook of Performing Arts Medicine*. New York, NY: Raven Press; 1991:319-336.
4. Pruett KD. Psychological aspects of the development of exceptionally young performers and prodigies. In: Sataloff RT, Brandfonbrener A, Lederman R, eds. *Textbook of Performing Arts Medicine*. New York, NY: Raven Press; 1991:337-350.

5. Rosen DC, Sataloff RT. Psychological aspects of voice disorders. In: Rubin JS, Sataloff RT, Korovin GS, Gould WJ, eds. *Diagnosis and Treatment of Voice Disorders.* New York, NY: Igaku Shoin Medical Publishers; 1995:491-501.
6. Shontz FC. Body image and physical disability. In: Cash TF, Pruzinsky, eds. *Body Images: Development Deviance and Change.* New York, NY: Guilford Press; 1990:157-169.
7. Freedman R. Cognitive behavioral perspectives on body image change. In: Cash TF, Pruzinsky, eds. *Body Images: Development Deviance and Change.* New York, NY: Guilford Press; 1990:273-295.
8. Stemple JC, Glaze LE, Gerdeman BK. *Clinical Voice Pathology: Theory and Management,* 2nd ed. San Diego, Calif: Singular Publishing Group Inc; 1995:255.

CHAPTER

9

Psychogenic Dysphonia

Voice disorders are divided into organic and nonorganic etiologies. Various terms have been used interchangeably (but imprecisely) to label observable vocal dysfunction in the presence of emotional factors that cause or perpetuate the symptoms. Stemple[1] describes the thorough documentation in the literature of the relationship of emotions to voice production and notes that references on this topic start as early as the middle 1800s with discussion of the need for emotional retraining and voice therapy. He refers the reader to Murphy, Brodnitz, Case, Colton, and Casper. Aronson argues convincingly for the term *psychogenic* which is "broadly synonymous with functional, but has the advantage of stating positively, based on an exploration of its causes, that the voice disorder is a manifestation of one or more types of psychological disequilibrium, such as anxiety, depression, conversion reaction, or personality disorder, that interfere with normal volitional control over phonation."[2(p121)]

Psychogenic disorders include a variety of discrete presentations. There is disagreement over classification among speech-language pathologists, with some excluding musculoskeletal tension disorders from this nomenclature. Aronson[2] and Butcher, Elias, and Raven[3] conclude that the hypercontraction of extrinsic and intrinsic laryngeal muscles, in response to emotional stress, is the "common denominator" behind the dysphonia or aphonia in these disorders. In addition, the extent of pathology visible on laryngeal examination is inconsistent with the severity of the abnormal voice. They cite four categories:

1. Musculoskeletal tension disorders: including vocal abuse, vocal nodules, contact ulcers, and ventricular dysphonia.
2. Conversion voice disorders: including conversion muteness and aphonia, conversion dysphonia, and psychogenic adductor "spasmodic dysphonia."
3. Mutational falsetto (puberphonia).
4. Childlike speech in adults.[2,3]

Psychogenic dysphonia may present as total inability to speak, whispered speech, extremely strained or strangled speech, interrupted speech rhythm, or speech in an abnormal register (such as falsetto in males after puberty). Usually, involuntary vocalizations during laughing and coughing are normal. The vocal folds are often difficult to examine because of supraglottic hyperfunction. There may be apparent bowing of both vocal folds due to severe muscular tension dysphonia creating anterior-posterior "squeeze" during phonation. Long-standing attempts to produce voice in the presence of this pattern may even result in traumatic lesions associated with vocal abuse patterns, such as vocal fold nodules. Normal abduction and adduction of the vocal folds may be visualized during flexible fiberoptic laryngoscopy by instructing the patient to perform maneuvers which decrease supraglottic "load," such as whistling or sniffing. In addition, the singing voice is often more easily produced than the speaking voice in these patients. Tongue extension by the laryngologist during the rigid telescopic portion of the examination often will result in clear voice. The severe muscular tension dysphonia associated with psychogenic dysphonia often can be eliminated by behavioral interventions by the speech-language pathologist, sometimes in one session. In some instances the laryngologist has been successful in restoring moments of normal voice during stroboscopic examination. According to the literature, psychogenic voice therapy focuses on modification of the emotional and psychosocial disturbances associated with the onset and maintenance of the voice problem. When the psychogenic causes are addressed and resolved, there usually will be resolution of the voice disorder.[1]

Laryngeal electromyography may be helpful in confirming the diagnosis by revealing simultaneous firing of abductors and adductors. Psychogenic dysphonia frequently has been misdiagnosed as spasmodic dysphonia, partially explaining the excellent "spasmodic dysphonia" cure rates in some series. Spasmodic dysphonia (SD) is considered by some researchers to be a neurologic syndrome and by others a symptom complex of multiple etiologies, neurologic and psychogenic. Sapir[4] argues that the debate over the etiology of spasmodic dysphonia can be resolved if spasmodic dysphonia is considered a neurologic syndrome and psychogenic spasmodic dysphonia a nonorganic phonatory disorder that mimics the syndrome, and if the voice symptoms and pathophysiologic characteristics of spasmodic dysphonia are well defined and agreed on. The authors reserve the term spasmodic laryngeal dysphonia for patients with neurogenic dystonia, although these patients frequently also display a secondary psychological response.

There is general consensus among physicians and speech-language pathologists that spasmodic dysphonia does not respond well to behavioral voice therapy. Differential diagnosis of neurologic and psychogenic voice disorders is most likely to be obtained through interdisciplinary collaboration between the laryngologist, neurologist, speech-language pathologist, and psychotherapist. This should include comprehensive medical assessment, including imaging studies, electrophysiologic testing, blood testing, and objective voice measures. Comprehensive assessment of vocal capabilities and impairments should be conducted by a speech-language pathologist with experience in treating this problem. A diagnostic interview by the psychological professional with regard to psychosocial, medical, and voice history with a view to their possible interrelationships should also be conducted early in the diagnostic process.[4] In his review of the literature, Sapir[4] notes that the neuropsychiatric database gives evidence for psychogenic motor disorders of many types, including dyskinesia, dystonia, myoclonus, tremor, ataxia, paresis, seizure, dysphonia, and dysarthria.

Psychogenic voice disorders are not merely the *absence* of observable neurolaryngeal abnormalities. This psychiatric diagnosis cannot be made with accuracy without the *presence* of a psychodynamic formulation based on understanding of the personality, motivations, conflicts, and primary as well as secondary gain associated with the symptoms. Butcher[5] and colleagues have summarized some etiologic factors in patients presenting with psychogenic voice disorders. These include an event of acute stress or prolonged anxiety, conflict over verbally expressing negative affect (particularly anger or resentment and personal opinions), predominance in female patients, lack of assertiveness accompanied by overcommitment and powerlessness, and otherwise minimal disruptions to psychological adjustment. Regardless of the precipitator, loss or impairment of the voice is a distressing experience for most patients, and their frustration and anger increase musculoskeletal tension and worsen vocal production.[5] Andrews[6] describes muscular "flight or fight" posturing of the laryngeal sphincter, as well as contribution from the intrinsic and extrinsic laryngeal musculature resulting from "life stressors, relational, and attitudinal conflicts."[(p382)] She further describes the characteristic communication style as the silent bearing of burdens, inadequate ventilation of feelings, the ethical manifesto to avoid complaint, and sublimation of their own needs and rights. Conversion disorders are a special classification of psychogenic symptomatology and reflect loss of voluntary control over striated muscle or the sensory systems as a reflection of stress or psychological conflict. This may occur in any organ system, but the target organ often is symbolically related to the specifics of the unconsciously perceived threat. The term was first used by Freud to describe a defense mechanism which rendered an intolerable wish or drive innocuous by translating its energy into a physical symptom. The presence of an ego-syntonic physical illness offers *primary gain*: relief from the anxiety, depression, or rage by maintaining the emotional conflict in the unconscious. *Secondary gain* often occurs by virtue of the "sick role."

Classic descriptions of findings in these patients include indifference to the symptoms, chronic stress, suppressed anger, immaturity and dependency, moderate depression, and poor sex role identification.[7,8] Conversion voice disorders also reflect a breakdown in communication with someone of emotional significance in the patient's life; wanting but blocking the verbal expression of anger, fear, or remorse; and significant feelings of shame.[2]

Confirmed neurological disease and psychogenic voice disorders do co-exist and are known as somatic compliance.[9,10] Of course, potential organic causes of psychiatric disorders must always be thoroughly investigated. Insidious onset of depression, personality changes, anxiety, or presumed conversion symptoms may be the first presentation of CNS disease.[11]

Psychological evaluation and psychotherapeutic management are the province of the mental health professional on the voice team. Ideally, this is an interdisciplinary, collaborative process. For treatment to be effective in the short-term and for treatment gains to persist, the psychosocial factors related to the voice disorder must be addressed. It matters very little whether they are causal or result from the voice disorder itself, but they must be addressed either directly or indirectly as part of the plan of care. Patients who exhibit severe emotional problems should be immediately referred to the psychological professional for assessment and treatment. However, complex, long-standing, and well-defended psychological conflicts may not be readily apparent.

Rogerian, client-centered counseling approaches in which the therapist is an attentive, empathic, and nonjudgmental listener are essential to the development of rapport in a therapeutic encounter between a clinician of any discipline and a patient. It is perfectly appropriate for professionals on the voice team to provide empathy, assist in the identification of concerns and their associated affect, and to integrate new insights about their feelings into communication strategies. However, graduate programs in speech-language pathology, vocal pedagogy, and theater do not, in general, provide psychological theory and clinical supervision to permit provision of psychotherapy that meets the current standard of care.[3] Voice professionals deserve treatment protocols in which the appropriate interventions are provided by the professional best educated to deliver them. It is the role of the psychological professional to help patients understand the psychosocial dynamics of vocal dysfunction. It would be unthinkable, for example, for the arts medicine psychologist to perform vocal fold surgery, and it is a questionable practice for most nonpsychiatrist physicians, nurses, speech-language pathologists, singing voice teachers, and acting voice specialists to assume that the inherently high level of empathy in most helping professions will be adequate to ensure proper psychological management.

Case Example: Psychogenic Dysphonia

Perhaps the most effective way to demonstrate the benefits of interdisciplinary care for patients with psychogenic voice disorders is by a case description. Major identifying features have been changed to provide protection of the patient's identity. "Mrs. G" was a woman in her early 60s when she first presented for evaluation and care at the voice center. She was accompanied during her evaluation by her husband who helped her to tell her story. She reported that she had been troubled by her whispered, strangled voice for approximately 1½ years and had had intermittent periods of total aphonia during that time. She had consulted a laryngologist near her home and, as a result, had had some psychotherapy with a psychiatrist.

She had been told that her voice difficulty was "psychosomatic." It dated to the events surrounding the death of one of her grandchildren 1½ years earlier while the child was in the care of the patient and her husband. The parents were away on a vacation at that time. The grandchild had had a long history of a treatment-resistant, chronic asthma and suffered status asthmaticus and subsequent respiratory arrest. CPR was instituted immediately and continuously administered, and the child was transported to a local emergency room. Attempts to resuscitate him failed. At the time of the child's death, the patient remained "in control" and "in charge." In the days and weeks which followed the funeral, she lapsed into the voice pattern observed during her evaluation. This was accompanied by pain on attempts to speak.

Mrs. G was unable to recount these events and, after the first sentence, began to cry silently. The remainder of the story was told by her husband. This patient responded with a full-blown panic attack when local anesthetic was administered to allow strobovideolaryngoscopic examination. The arts medicine psychologist accompanied the patient to the examination room, and behavioral and cognitive strategies were employed to control the episode of panic. Her strobovideolaryngoscopic findings were consistent with severe muscular tension dysphonia.

During her evaluation by the speech-language pathologist, the patient volunteered a particularly descriptive and potent metaphor. This was reflected back to her with great empathy by the speech-language pathologist, and the patient began to sob uncontrollably. This broke the pattern of high chest breathing which she had been employing throughout the interview. She reported that the prior psychotherapist had assured her that the comparatively brief period of psychotherapy was customary for the facilitation of grief work.

This patient was referred for ongoing treatment with the author (DCR) as an adjunct to her work with the voice team and the remainder of her medical evaluation. A number of relevant issues emerged. This patient demonstrated the features typical of a psychogenic voice disorder. She had a history of being the "broad shouldered," competent, stabilizing individual within her extended family. Her father had deserted the family during her early adolescence, and her own mother had "borne up in dignity and in silence." Her therapy allowed for opportunities, through enactment, to finally express the unspoken feelings to both her father and mother. Her own marriage was characterized by a pattern of verbal deference to her husband, while handling and diffusing family crises and dilemmas out of his view.

Her son and daughter-in-law, parents of the dead child, became withdrawn and aloof as a result of their own grief. They were unable to tolerate an account of the events leading up to and immediately following the child's death. The patient was tormented by her fantasies that they held her to blame for an inadequate response to the child's mortal event and that they could no longer trust the patient with the care of any of their other children. This was particularly painful since, for this patient, her children and grandchildren were the center of her life. Finally, the dead child's siblings and cousins turned to her for opportunities to discuss and describe their feelings, positive and negative, toward him. This expression of emotion and need for information was discouraged by the children's parents. So, it needed to be conducted in secret and presented conflict for the patient in respecting the parents' authority. She had enormous "unfinished business" with the dead child himself.

Therapeutic sessions focused on the historical reasons for silence, lack of assertiveness, and the patient's split of her "good and bad" selves. She was assisted to communicate more openly with her husband during couples' sessions and encouraged to support the extended family in family therapy interventions to allow grief resolution for them. Referrals were made to excellent family therapists in the patient's locale. Finally, the patient finished her grief work using a variety of verbal and nonverbal modalities of expression. She learned to value her communicative self, and to honor her expressions of love and grief. Her voice returned to normal, and her vocal complaints have not recurred.

REFERENCES

1. Stemple J, Glaze L, Goldman B. *Clinical Voice Pathology: Theory and Management,* 2nd ed. San Diego, Calif: Singular Publishing Group Inc; 1995:169.
2. Aronson, A. *Clinical Voice Disorders,* 3rd ed. New York, NY: Thieme Medical Publishers; 1990:117-145.
3. Butcher P, Elias A, Raven R. *Psychogenic Voice Disorders and Cognitive-Behavior Therapy.* San Diego, Calif: Singular Publishing Group Inc; 1993:3-22.
4. Sapir S. Psychogenic spasmodic dysphonia: a case setting with expert opinions. *J Voice.* 9:270-281.
5. Butcher P, Elias A, Raven R. *Psychogenic Voice Disorders and Cognitive Behavior Therapy.* London: Whurr Publishers Ltd; 1993:9-11.
6. Andrews M. *Manual of Voice Treatment: Pediatrics Through Geriatrics.* San Diego, Calif: Singular Publishing Group Inc; 1995:380-389.
7. Nemiah J. Psychoneurotic disorders. In: Nicholi A, ed. *The New Harvard Guide to Psychiatry.* Cambridge, MA: Harvard University Press; 1988:234-258.
8. Ziegler FS, Imboden JB. Contemporary conversion reactions: II. conceptual model. *Arch Gen Psychiatry.* 1962;6:279-287.
9. Sapir S, Aronson A. Coexisting psychogenic and neurogenic dysphonia: a source of diagnostic confusion. *Br J Disord Com.* 1987;22:73-80.
10. Hartman D, Daily W, Morin K. A case of superior laryngeal nerve paresis and psychogenic dysphonia. *J Speech Hearing Disord.* 1989;54:526-529.
11. Cummings J, Benson D, Houlihan J, Gosenfield L. Mutism: loss of neocortical and limbic vocalization. *J Nerv Ment Dis.* 1983;171:255-259.

CHAPTER

10

Response to Vocal Injury

"To sing is to be." (Rilke) So states the quotation which hangs on the wall near my desk (DCR), and the quotation is apt when the music making is going well. When it is not, the opposite view, not to sing is not to be, holds significant psychological peril for the serious voice student and professional singer. The impact is very similar for professional actors and other professional speakers.

In all of us, self-esteem comprises not only who we believe we are, but also what we believe we do: a double exposure exists then for performers who cannot separate these two elements of performance. Unlike the instrumentalist whose artistry is an interplay between the musician and the instrument, or even the actor whose craft encompasses almost equally a myriad of elements of performance, the singer's voice is (or is often perceived to be) everything. The voice is in, is therefore of, indeed *is* the self. The goal of the psychological professional working collaboratively with the voice injured professional voice user is to disarticulate the "self" as vessel for the voice from the sense of self as the voice, which is so replete with psychological danger for the injured performer. The psychotherapist must gradually reintroduce all the properties that comprise self definition and, therefore, provide for a full and meaningful life as he or she assists the individual to achieve emotional balance. For many performers, this is painfully difficult.

Before beginning to explore the psychological impact of vocal injury, it may be useful, for theoretical clarity, to divide the experience of vocal injury into several phases. In practice, however, they often overlap or recur, and the emotional responses are not entirely linear.

1. *The phase of problem recognition:* The patient "feels" that "something" is wrong, but may not be able to clearly define the problem, especially if the onset has been gradual or masked by a co-existing illness. Usually, personal "first-aid" measures will be tried, and when they fail, the performer will manifest some level of panic. This often is followed by feelings of guilt when the distress is turned inward against the self, or rage/blame when externalized.

2. *The phase of diagnosis:* This may be a protracted period if an injured performer does not have immediate access to a laryngologist experienced in the assessment of vocal injury. He or she may have already consulted with voice teachers, family physicians, allergists, nutritionists, peers, or otolaryngologists and speech-language pathologists without specialized training in caring for professional voice users. There may have been several, possibly contradictory, diagnoses and treatment protocols. The vocal dysfunction persists, and the patient grows more fearful and discouraged. If attempts to perform are continued, they may exacerbate the injury and/or produce embarrassing performances. The fear is of the unknown, but it is intuitively perceived as significant.

3. *Phase of treatment: Acute/rehabilitative:* Fear of the unknown becomes fear of the known and of its outcome. The performer, now in the "sick role," initially feels overwhelmed, powerless, and vulnerable. There is frequently a strong component of blame which may be turned inward. "Why me, why now?" is the operant, recurrent thought. Vocal rehabilitation is an exquisitely slow, carefully monitored, often frustrating process, and many patients become fearful and impatient. Some will meet the criteria for major depression, which will be discussed in additional detail, as will the impact of vocal fold surgery.

4. *Phase of acceptance:* When the acute and rehabilitative treatment protocol is complete, the final prognosis is clearer. When there are significant lasting changes in the voice, the patient will experience mourning. Even when there is full return of vocal function, a sense of vulnerability lingers. These individuals are likely to adhere strictly, even ritualistically, to preventive vocal hygiene habits and may be anxious enough to become hypochondriacal.[1]

The threat to body image and, consequently, self-image that can arise when an individual is confronted with any medical problem has been well researched. According to Freud, the ego is first and foremost a body ego, and the ego defenses, which are unconscious, serve to protect the individual by distorting reality and thus reducing anxiety. The use of the compensation defenses (projection, reaction formation), regression, and repression can be readily seen in patients struggling to maintain emotional equilibrium after the trauma of a significant medical diagnosis.[2] Later researchers such as Schilder,[3] Fenichel,[4] and Blum, et al[5] expanded Freud's theoretical conceptions by recognizing that body image is dynamic and responds to both internal experience and social forces.

The self-concept is an essential construct of Carl Rodgers' theories of counseling. Rodgers described self-concept as composed of perceptions of the characteristics of the self and the relationships of the self to various aspects of life, as well as the values attached to the perceptions.[6] Rodgers suggested that equilibrium requires that patients' self-concepts be congruent with their life experiences. It follows, then, that it is not the disability per se that psychologically influences the person, but rather the subjective meaning and feelings attached to the disability. According to Rodgers, the two major psychological defenses which operate to maintain consistent self-concept are denial and distortion.[6]

Kurt Lewin's[7] *field theory* is social-psychological in nature. It stresses the importance of contemporaneity, that is, the idea that behavior can best be understood in its immediate manifestations and by understanding the individual in relationship to his or her larger environment. Lewin's theory has stimulated significant theoretical work in conceptualizing the psychological effects of any physical disability. Lewin, and later researchers of his theory, also stress that it is the personal meaning of the disability, in conjunction with the stimulus value that that disability holds for others in the patient's life space, that is important in understanding the psychological adjustment the patient makes to the disability itself.[7]

The majority of research in this area has examined reactions to loss of the special senses (hearing and vision), loss of a body part (mastectomy, amputation), and the consequence of life-threatening illness (cancer, heart disease). The theoretical underpinnings for this work depend heavily on research which has been done on grief and mourning after death of a loved one and the body of psychophysiological research on stress responses. Review of the relevant literature has revealed very little with regard to the impact of loss of voice as it is defined *by the voice user* and its psychological consequences. The literature in speech-language pathology describes manifestations and supportive interventions for patients demonstrating maladaptive psychological adjustment after laryngectomy, laryngeal trauma, and gender-inappropriate voice quality.[8-11]

Reaction to illness is the major source of psychiatric disturbance in patients with significant voice dysfunction. Loss of communicative function is an experience of alienation which threatens human self-definition and independence. Catastrophic fears of loss of productivity, economic and social status, and creative artistry in professional voice users contribute to rising anxiety. Anxiety is known to worsen existing

communication disorders, and the disturbances in memory, concentration, and synaptic transmission secondary to depression may intensify
other voice symptoms and interfere with rehabilitation. Families of patients are affected, as well. They are often confused about the diagnosis
and poorly prepared to support the patient's coping responses. The resulting stress may negatively influence family dynamics and intensify
the depressive illness.[12]

Essentially, the patient with a voice injury goes through a grieving
process similar to patients who mourn for other losses. In a significant
number of cases, especially among voice professionals, the patients actually mourn the loss of their "self" as they perceive it. Losses vary in
terms of how significant they are. No one can properly determine the
significance of any particular loss to someone else. The significance of a
loss depends on the intensity of the attachment, the number of related
losses, and the extent to which the patient's daily routine or habits are
disrupted. Therefore, the first step in comprehending the loss concept
is to analyze the importance of the event to the particular patient. In the
truest of psychological senses, it is the emotional meaning the particular object has for the individual that is all-important and will predict
the type of reaction which will follow its loss.

It is important to remember that the loss of an object may be threatened or actual, symbolic or fantasized. According to the work of Hislop,[14] and Joffe and Sandler,[15] a fundamental factor determining the
outcome of loss is the nature of the relationship that previously existed;
specifically, whether there has been love for and need for the lost object
and what it represents. If the lost object has been needed, it has been an
essential part of the person's self-support system. If the presence of the
lost object is essential for approximating the actual to the ideal self, its
loss will inevitably result in distress. This is fundamental to the understanding of grief: there exists an intense feeling of some integral loss of
self.[13-15]

As the voice-injured patient experiences the process of grieving,
the psychologist may assume a more prominent role in his or her care.
The psychological professional is responsible for facilitating the tasks of
mourning and monitoring the individual's formal mental status for
clinically significant changes. Lazare estimates that 10%–15% of people
who pass through the mental health clinics at Massachusetts General
Hospital have, underlying their psychiatric diagnosis, an unresolved
grief reaction.[16]

Losses have the potential for both growth and regression, and there
is extensive evidence that losses can have negative, even disastrous,
consequences. These consequences have a number of manifestations.
Unresolved loss makes it less likely that subsequent losses will be re-

solved, and the failure of grief resolution keeps emotional energy bound to the past and to the loss. Significant loss affects people physically and enhances their vulnerability to subsequent illness.[13] It also disrupts the emotional well-being of the individual by confronting him or her with intrusive and painfully difficult emotions.[13] Loss deprives people of their sense of security because one significant loss serves to remind them of how fragile their control over what happens really is. Therefore, an actual loss is also a threat of other potential losses and may make the future a source of fear as it becomes painfully clear that predictability is merely a fantasy.[13]

The definition of grief developed by Rando applies particularly well to the responses professional voice users make to perceived or actual loss of the voice as they know it. *Grief* refers to the process of experiencing the psychological, social, and physical reactions to one's perception of loss. Grief is a continuing development and involves many changes over time. It is also a natural and expected reaction to all kinds of losses. *Mourning* consists of the conscious and unconscious processes that gradually undo the psychological ties to the lost object, assist in adaptation to this loss, and make it possible to live fully in a world without it.[17,18]

There are a number of models for tracking this process. The most easily understood is that of Worden, as adapted by the author (DCR). The patient accomplishes the tasks of mourning while moving through three major phases of response.[18,19] Grief work is not an orderly and unvarying process, and it seldom progresses forward without fluctuation. The responses of grievers also are quite personal and are influenced by a variety of individual characteristics and psychological, social, and physical factors. The major phases are *avoidance* in which there is shock, denial, and disbelief; *confrontation*, the state in which one learns that the loss is permanent and the psychological, physical, and spiritual responses are most acute; and *accommodation* during which there is a gradual decline of acute grief and the beginning of an emotional and social reentry into a world in which the lost object no longer exists.[17]

The initial task is to *accept the reality of the loss*. The need for and distress of this is vestigial during the phase of diagnosis in the professional voice user, is held consciously in abeyance during the acute and rehabilitative phases of treatment, but is reenforced with accumulating data measuring vocal function. As the reality becomes undeniable, the mourner must be helped to express the full range of grieving affect. The rate of accomplishing this is variable and individual. Generally, it will occur in the style with which the person usually copes with crisis and may be quite florid or tightly constricted. All responses must be invited and normalized. The psychologist facilitates the process and stays particularly attuned to unacceptable, split-off responses or the failure to move through any particular response.

As attempts to deny the loss take place and fail, the mourner gradually encounters the next task: *beginning to live and cope in a world in which the lost object is absent.* This is the psychoanalytic process of *decathexis*, requiring the withdrawal of life energies from the other and the reinvesting of them in the self. For some professional voice users, this may be a temporary state as they make adjustments required by their rehabilitation demands. In other cases, the need for change will be lasting; change in fach, change in repertoire, need for amplification, altered performance schedule, or, occasionally, change in career.

As the patient so injured seeks to heal his or her life, another task demand looms. Known as *recathexis*, it involves *reinvesting life energies in other relationships, interests, talents, and life goals.*[1,19]

Grieving a loss to successful resolution implies that the mourner has been able to abstract meaning from something that initially seemed meaningless. An event in life which the patient did not and would not ever choose actually had positive outcomes, led to greater self-motivation, and provided a greater sense of personal freedom than ever before. Resolving losses in this way involves relinquishing the customary cognitive set, which views the personal loss as tragic and limiting, and replacing it with a reformulation of the experience in terms of opportunities, possibilities, and growth.[13] Morris West describes this process in *Shoes of the Fisherman:* "One has to abandon altogether the search for security, and reach out to the risk of living with both arms. One has to embrace the world like a lover. One has to accept pain as a condition of existence. One has to court doubt and darkness as the cost of knowing. One needs a will stubborn in conflict, but apt always to total acceptance of every consequence of living and dying."[20(p117)] Rosen and Sataloff have written that many of the overwhelmingly disabling responses of professional voice users to permanent voice change could be avoided from the outset by development of an appropriate perspective, a well-rounded education that involves more than just voice, and healthy respect for the worth of one's self separate from the all-important voice.[1]

Professional voice users with significant lasting changes in vocal quality or stamina experience a serious threat to self-definition and self-image. When the change is permanent, they must acknowledge and grieve the loss of a body part and release the associated negative emotions. When the progress is uncertain, vocal professionals will move through several phases of emotional adjustment which necessitate reality testing and appropriately tailored psychological interventions.

A preliminary, previously unpublished research study using the case study method has helped clarify these responses. Common psychological characteristics of the patients and their cognitive, affective, and behavioral presentation relative to their phase of vocal injury were evaluated. Subjects were drawn from patients referred to our medical practice specializing in the care of the voice. Following an existing protocol, they were medically evaluated, including assessment by strobovideolaryngoscopy, objective voice measures to document baseline vocal pathology, and assessment by the various professionals of the voice treatment team. Informed consent regarding the limits of confidentiality in that setting was obtained by the author.

Patients were interviewed in: (1) the phase of diagnosis, (2) the phase of treatment, acute/rehabilitative, and (3) the phase of acceptance. A psychological evaluation, including relevant psychiatric and psychosocial history and current mental status, was conducted. Of specific interest were current and cumulative psychological stressors, especially losses and significant changes in lifestyle. Coping responses to perceived voice impairment in the selected population were identified and revealed signs and symptoms of classic grief reaction. A number of self-report measures were also administered during each contact with the research subjects. Expressive, projective documentation was obtained through the use of self-portrait and artistic representations of "the voice" at each session, as well.

Although the number of subjects who completed all components of the research protocol was too small for valid statistical inference, the self-report materials and responses to structured questions during the clinical interview reflect psychological progression through the phases associated with grief in the literature. The artwork provided fascinating windows into self-perception and the patient's body awareness with regard to laryngeal function. Some of these cases are presented in descriptive form in Chapter 17.

Participation in the research itself, especially the completion of materials that highlighted the physical, affective, cognitive, and behavioral manifestations of grief, normalized these responses and produced a marked decrease in patient anxiety. The structured clinical interviews provided an opportunity for the release of grieving affect and catharsis, especially of anger turned outward toward the members of the voice treatment team and inward as guilt. Finally, reformulation of the meaning of the vocal injury in terms of opportunity took place in almost every research subject. Patients universally spoke of the "rehearsal" for disappointment provided by the rigorous and competitive experiences of professional vocal training. This also is consistent with research on stress inoculation and the outcome of resolution of prior, less threatening losses.

As a certified professional grief counsellor, the author (DCR) has long had a subspecialty in grief and loss counseling in her clinical practice. The literature provides a great many creative, useful models of grief counseling for those individuals experiencing uncomplicated mourning, and grief therapy for those in whom grief reactions have become pathological. A variety of these modalities are described in Chapter 15 on psychotherapeutic techniques.

REFERENCES

1. Rosen DC, Sataloff RT, Evans H, Hawkshaw M. Self-esteem in singers: singing healthy, singing hurt. *NATS J.* 1993;49:32-35.
2. Freud S. *The Ego and the Id.* London: Hogarth Press; 1927:31-35.
3. Schilder P. *The Image and Appearance of the Human Body.* London: Paul Keegan Press; 1935.
4. Fenichel O. *The Psychoanalytic Theory of Neurosis.* New York, NY: W.W. Norton; 1945.
5. Blum G, Barley G, Guffels C. The concept of body image and the remediation of body image disorders. *J Learning Dis.* 1970;3:440-447.
6. Rodgers CR. A theory of therapy, personality, and interpersonal relationships as developed in a client-centered framework. In: Koch S, ed. *Psychology: A Study of a Science,* New York, NY: McGraw-Hill Book Company; 1959;3:184-256.
7. Lewin K. *A Dynamic Theory of Personality.* New York, NY: McGraw-Hill Book Company; 1935:130.
8. Stemple J, Glaze L, Gerdeman B. *Clinical Voice Pathology: Theory and Management,* 2nd ed. San Diego, Calif: Singular Publishing Group, Inc; 1995:167-228, 270-326.
9. Andrews M. *Manual of Voice Treatment: Pediatrics Through Geriatrics.* San Diego, Calif: Singular Publishing Group Inc; 1995.
10. Aronson A. *Clinical Voice Disorders,* 3rd ed. New York, NY: Thieme Medical Publishers; 1990.
11. Boone D. *The Voice and Voice Therapy.* Englewood Cliffs, CA: Prentice-Hall Publishers; 1971.
12. Zraick R, Boone D. Spouse attitudes toward a person with aphasia. *J Speech Hear Res.* 1991;34:123-128.
13. Schneider J. Stress, *Loss, and Grief: Understanding Their Origins and Growth Potential.* Rockville, MD: Aspen Systems Corporation; 1984:28-33, 208-220.
14. Hislop I. *Stress, Distress, and Illness.* Sydney: McGraw-Hill Book Company; 1991:9-17.
15. Joffe WG, Sandler J. Notes on pain, depression, and individuation. *Psychoanalytic Study of the Child.* 1965;20:394-424.
16. Lazare A. Unresolved grief. In: Lazare A, ed. *Outpatient Psychiatry: Diagnosis and Treatment.* Baltimore, MD: Williams and Wilkins; 1979:498-512.

17. Rando T. *Grief, Dying, and Death: Clinical Interventions for Care-Givers.* New York, NY: Research Press; 1984.
18. Rando T. *Grieving: How to Go on Living When Someone You Love Dies.* Lexington, Mass: Lexington Books; 1988:11-24.
19. Worden JW. *Grief Counselling and Grief Therapy: A Handbook for the Mental Health Practitioner.* New York, NY: Springer Publishing Company; 1982:7-34.
20. West M. *Shoes of the Fisherman,* New York, NY: William Morrow and Company; 1963:117.

CHAPTER

11

Response to Voice Surgery

When vocal fold surgery is indicated, many individuals will demonstrate hospital-related phobias or self-destructive responses to pain. Adamson et al describe the importance of understanding how the patient's occupational identity will be affected by surgical intervention.[1] Vocal fold surgery impacts on the major mode of communication utilized by all human beings. Even temporary periods of absolute voice rest (silence) which may be necessary following surgery may induce feelings of insecurity, helplessness, and dissociation from the verbal world. In professional voice users, the psychological exposure is increased and intensified. The predominant presenting symptoms are most likely to be mood disturbance and/or significant anxiety. Psychological variables, especially those of a cognitive nature, are related to many of the adjustment and recovery problems encountered in health care delivery; and these variables are important factors in planning psychological interventions.[2]

Most adults facing surgery for any reason experience fears of pain, mutilation, possible death, uncertainty about the outcome, and feelings of helplessness. "Effective problems solvers" demonstrate less depression, less psychosocial impairment, and greater assertiveness in populations of patients with severe physical disabilities.[3] Patients make inferences about their physiological states and sensations, and some people are more prone to interpret these sensations as symptomatic of physical illness; whereas others are more conservative and logical in their interpretations. This underlies the theoretical value of problem-solving appraisal.

Individuals also differ in their beliefs about the impact of their behavior on actual health outcomes, their desire for information about health-related issues, and the degree to which they want to be directly involved in their own health care. These preferences can have a substantial impact on the level of individual distress prior to enduring medical and surgical procedures.[3] A proper surgical discussion highlights vocal fold surgery as elective. The patient chooses surgery as the only remaining means to try to recover a "normal voice" or a different, but more desirable, voice. The laryngologist and entire voice team must understand the motivations for this choice of treatment modality and how the motivations relate to the patient's subjective body image and its emotional and interpersonal context.[4]

Responsible care includes a thorough documented, preoperative discussion of the limits and complications of surgery, with recognition by the surgeon that anxiety affects both understanding and retention of information about undesirable outcomes. According to Prugh and Thompson, very high degrees of narcissistic involvement in a particular body part can lead to psychological problems that endure after surgical healing is complete.[5] In less psychologically impaired patients who are undergoing restorative procedures, assimilation of body image change is unlikely to be significantly disruptive. What is "restored" exists in the memory stores of the patient's experience.[4] Personality psychopathology or unrealistic expectations of the impact of surgery on their lives are elements for which surgical candidates can be screened. When surgery is technically successful but does not match the patient's conception of the outcome, patients will often react very negatively.[4,6,7] Recognizing such problems preoperatively allows preoperative counseling and obviates many postoperative difficulties. Carpenter[8] details the value of an early therapy session to focus on the fears, fantasies, misconceptions, and regression that frequently accompany a decision to undergo surgery.

Postoperative psychological care may entail individual or group counseling for patients whose psychological distress appears out of proportion to the vocal pathology and its treatment course. Postoperative changes in self-perception, cognition, emotion, and voicing behaviors do not occur immediately after release of restrictions of voice use. A period of vocal rehabilitation is usually a component of surgical management. There may well be an initial exacerbation in the emotion, time, and attention given to the voice and significant anxiety about audible changes in vocal quality. This is not unexpected, and psychological professionals are aware that, when important psychological change occurs, there is often a period of emotional disequilibrium. Patients who are able to experience and tolerate this moderate level of emotional disruption are more likely to experience major, positive therapeutic benefits.

Referrals will often be made to the psychological professional on the voice team when the patient continues to manifest depression and dissatisfaction with his or her life and vocal quality in spite of technically excellent surgical results. Of particular concern are patients who cannot integrate the objectively validated return to "normal voice." They are similar to "insatiable" plastic surgery patients who repeatedly request cosmetic surgery, often multiple surgical procedures on the same body parts. Research on this patient population has revealed the presence of borderline personality organization with characteristic general instability and a psychological identity that includes body image diffuseness.[9] Research on the causes of patient dissatisfaction with the results of technically satisfactory surgery by MacGregor[6] revealed elements such as patient psychopathology and unrealistic expectations of the surgical correction on their lives. Dissatisfaction also was noted to occur if the surgeon had not explained the nature of the surgery in terms that the patient could understand.

Many postoperative difficulties can be alleviated if patients receive support from a therapist for normal feelings of anxiety, sadness, and frustration. Both individual and group treatment can allow an integration of problem-solving strategies and specific self-management and stress management interventions. Specifically, patients may be taught the use of emotion-focused strategies such as imagery and relaxation exercises. Auerbach[2] has recommended these strategies as particularly efficacious in assisting patients in regulating emotional experiences of brief duration over which the patient has little actual control.

A case example follows which illustrates a preoperative patient whose underlying psychological issues made her a poor surgical risk. Short-term therapeutic interventions were designed based on a diagnostic assessment. These allowed the patient to resolve phobic responses based on past trauma and obtain satisfactory affective and behavioral control to permit vocal fold surgery.

PREPARATION FOR SURGERY

This patient was a contemporary Christian singer in her early thirties who also composed much of her own music and accompanied herself. She had sought diagnosis and treatment from a number of otolaryngologists prior to travelling to the voice center for assessment and care. At the time of her examination, strobovideolaryngoscopy revealed the presence of vocal fold masses and evidence of prior vocal fold hemorrhage. Muscle tension dysphonia and compensatory, improper singing voice technique were also noted. The patient underwent a period of intensive voice therapy during which these compensatory patterns were eliminated. She was scheduled to undergo surgery for excision of the vocal fold mass, but expressed significant anxiety, bordering on panic, to her surgeon during a preoperative examination. She was referred to the arts medicine psychologist for assessment and preparation for surgery.

Patients who are in a state of physiologic hyperarousal and who describe premonitions of poor outcome from anesthesia or surgery are classified as poor surgical risks. This patient had travelled to the center from another state and was without the usual support system upon which she depended. She had been praying actively for guidance that this was "the right path" for her to pursue in order to return to her ministry through music. She felt that she had not gotten a clear "sign" that she should proceed.

In exploring her fears, the patient revealed that she had undergone gynecologic surgery as an adolescent and had experienced postoperative complications which were treated, but resulted in impairment of her fertility. The patient and her husband were actively engaged in attempting to conceive a child, and the medical interventions necessary to this process were experienced as intrusive, undignified, and distressing. This woman had experienced a classical conditioning response of anxiety and negative expectations to the surgical experience. In addition, the nature of the surgery for gynecologic problems occurred at a developmentally sensitive time and was perceived, emotionally, as an assault. The unfortunate consequent infertility was a source of enormous sadness to the patient and her husband, and the necessary infertility treatments were interfering with her experience of the privacy and sacredness of the process of conception.

She had developed a phobic response to anesthesia and the "invasion" of any body orifice. She was significantly ambivalent about the upcoming voice surgery for two reasons: First, she feared the loss of control inherent in surgery and the lack of any absolute promise of a perfect outcome, and although she trusted the laryngologist, he represented another "invading male." Second, the patient wished intensely to become pregnant and have a child, and had wondered intermittently whether she could conduct her performing career and adequately mother at the same time. She had just completed her first CD and had been offered a contract for a second recording.

Progressive relaxation was taught, practiced, and anchored tactilely using a touch on the shoulder from the therapist to enter a state of deep relaxation. Once both patient and therapist were satisfied that this could be successfully accomplished, the neurolinguistic programming (NLP) technique of "collapsing anchors" was used for elements of the early adolescent surgical experience. These elements were collected with the patient in a dissociated state of memory, observing herself in the scene and describing the sensory elements to the therapist who recorded them on a chalk board as a further means of maintaining the dissociation. A memory of safety, well-being, and relaxation was evoked and anchored to the same spot used for the progressive muscle relaxation exercise. The patient was then returned to the prior negative experience in an associated fashion, taking with her the positive visual, auditory, kinesthetic, olfactory, and gustatory experiences which had been anchored as previously described. Emergence was conducted, and the patient and therapist discussed the adequacy of this experience. The patient expressed disbelief that she could no longer recover the formerly negative responses, even when she was instructed to try to do so.

The patient and the therapist then conducted a search for those elements which would be necessary for the patient to feel safe and to "have a sign" that her voice surgery was in the best interests of her life plan. These were enumerated, and prior experiences in the patient's life that contained these elements were recalled, reexperienced, and anchored in an altered state. These anchors were "stacked" until both the patient and the therapist were comfortable that they were adequately potent. Induction was conducted, and the patient was invited to create a future fantasy image of herself in the anesthesia preparation area and the operating room for her vocal fold surgery. She was invited to maintain the degree of awareness that would allow her to observe the scene and herself in it (in imagery) with final, authoritative "emergency veto power" at any point during the surgery. She was then instructed to observe the events as they unfolded from the time of her arrival in the anesthesia preparation area to her return visit to the voice center for her immediate post-op visit and clearance to return home. She did so in the state of deep trance, and felt no need to exercise her "veto power." The psychologist then assisted the patient in firing the stacked anchor in a awake state. Fractionalized induction to deep trance was conducted, and suggestions were given that she could fire this anchor when she arrived in the anesthesia preparation area and "enjoy all the benefits of this deeply relaxed state of mind and pleasantly and comfortably awaken in the postanesthesia care unit or in your own hospital room." The patient chose to undergo vocal fold surgery which proceeded uneventfully. The healing was complete, and the patient has returned to her performing career. She is also the mother of an infant.

REFERENCES

1. Adamson JD, Hersuberg D, Shane F. The psychic significance of parts of the body in surgery. In: Howells JG, ed. *Modern Perspectives in the Psychiatric Aspects of Surgery*. New York, NY: Brunner Mazel; 1976:20-45.
2. Auerbach SM. Stress management and coping research in the health care setting: an overview and methological commentary. *J Consult Clin Psych.* 1989;57:388-395.
3. Elliott TR, Marmarosh CL. Problem solving appraisal: health complaints and health-related expectancies. *J Counsel Devel.* 1994;72:531-537.
4. Pruzinsky T, Edgerton M. Body image change in plastic surgery. In: Cash T, Pruzinsky T, eds. *Body Images: Development, Deviance, and Change*. New York, NY: The Guilford Press; 1990:217-236.
5. Prugh DG, Thompson TL. Illness as a source of stress: acute illness, chronic illness, and surgical procedures. In: Nospitz J, Coppington R, eds. *Stressors and the Adjustment Disorders*. New York, NY: John Wiley and Sons; 1990.
6. MacGregor SC. Patients' dissatisfaction with results of technically satisfactory surgery. *Aesthet Plast Surg.* 1981;5:27-32.
7. Shontz F. Body image and physical disability. In: Cash T, Pruzinsky T, eds. *Body Images: Development, Deviance, and Change*. New York, NY: The Guilford Press; 1990:149-169.
8. Carpenter B. Psychological aspects of vocal fold surgery. In: Gould WJ, Sataloff RT, Spiegel JR, eds. *Voice Surgery*. St. Louis, Mo: Mosby Year-Book Inc; 1993:339-343.
9. Groenman NH, Sauer HC. Personality characteristics of the cosmetic surgical insatiable patient. *Psychother Psychosomat.* 1983;40:241-245.

CHAPTER

12

Response to Neurologic Disorders Affecting Communication

atients with neurological disease commonly experience psychiatric symptoms, especially depression and anxiety. These disorders cause physiologic change which may exacerbate or mask the underlying neurologic presentation. Metcalfe and colleagues cite the incidence of severe depression and/or anxiety in neurologic patients at one-third.[1] Site of lesion affects the incidence, with lesions of the left cerebral hemisphere, basal ganglia, limbic system, thalamus, and anterior frontal lobe more likely to produce depression and anxiety.[2] The same structures are important in voice, speech, and language production. So, depression and anxiety logically coexist with voice and language disorders resulting from central nervous system (CNS) pathology.[2,3] Many voice symptoms are present in a wide range of neurological disorders. Aronson reviewed dysphonias associated with neurological disease in 1980 and reported that neurologic voice disorders are technically dysarthrias and are most often found in concert with a "complex of respiratory, resonatory, and articulatory dysarthric signs."[4(p71)]

Stemple summarizes neurological disorders with associated voice symptoms and organizes them by site-of-lesion, including: (1) the upper motor neurons, (2) the extra-pyramidal system, (3) the cerebellum, (4) the lower motor neurons, and (5) the peripheral nervous system and myoneural junction.[5] The psychological professional is referred to neuroanatomy and neurophysiology texts to review the impact of damage to central nervous system tissue and the sensory and motor pathways of the nervous system that innervate respiratory, phonatory, and articulatory muscles. The presentation of disruption will depend on the site of lesion and degree of damage, and may well affect respiratory, swallowing, and/or vocal production. Psychological professionals who accept responsibility for the care of patients with these disorders must familiarize themselves with the impact of each of these types of pathology on activities of daily living. This is critical in assisting these patients to live behaviorally and emotionally adaptive lives within the limits of their diseases.

Vocal fold paralysis may be unilateral or bilateral, central or peripheral, and it may involve the recurrent laryngeal nerve, superior laryngeal nerve, or both.[6] The laryngologist will confirm suspected vocal fold paralysis visually, radiographically, and electromyographically in order to plan appropriate treatment to protect the airway and improve vocal quality. Vocal fold paralysis may be caused by viral illness, tumor, or trauma (including surgery) and various other factors which must be investigated. The true incidence of vocal fold paralysis remains unknown.[7] Patients with unilateral vocal fold paralysis will be referred to speech-language pathologists for assessment, including identification of compensatory behaviors which are counter-productive. The speech-language pathologist provides patients with education about vocal hygiene and specific therapeutic modalities directed toward progressive development of optimal breathing, abdominal support, and intrinsic laryngeal muscle strength and agility. When the patient has complied with voice therapy, improvement has reached a plateau, and patients feel that their voice quality is still not satisfactory for their purposes, surgery may be indicated. A variety of surgical interventions is available, and the reader is directed to Chapter 4 on medical and surgical management of voice disorders in this textbook and to the many additional references cited therein. When vocal fold paralysis is bilateral, there is still no satisfactory treatment. These patients may have to decide, in collaboration with their physicians, between the options of good voice and tracheotomy, or good airway and bad voice.[6]

Dysphonia is voice disturbance, usually at the level of the larynx, and dysarthria refers to imperfect speech articulation.[6] This condition is actually symptomatic of any one of a group of disorders that affects strength, speed, and coordination, and involves the brain, as well as the nerves and musculature of the mouth, larynx, and respiratory system as they relate to speech. Dysarthria may be the first sign of a serious neurological problem noticed by professional voice users, because of their careful scrutiny of vocal production.[6]

Dysarthria may result from vascular, metabolic, motor, traumatic, or infectious causes; and it may be acute or progressive (slowly or rapidly). Patients who exhibit dysarthria will be evaluated jointly by a laryngologist, neurologist, and speech-language pathologist to establish a cause and provide the most appropriate treatment. Speech therapy will be essential in helping these patients maintain intelligible communication for as long as possible. Psychological professionals who provide adjunctive care to these patients must work closely with the patients' speech-language pathologist and understand the treatment plan and communication strategies. These can be reinforced during therapy sessions and will strengthen the behavioral conditioning responses.

Parkinson's disease, a progressive movement disorder, is characterized by decrease in spontaneous movement, gait difficulty, postural instability, rigidity, and resting tremor. It is caused by degeneration of the substantia nigra resulting in decreased dopamine availability. The primary etiology of Parkinson's disease has not been determined. Psychological professionals are familiar with extra-pyramidal symptoms since they are side effects of some psychoactive medications. Depression has been reported in approximately 30% of patients with Parkinson's disease; and as the disease progresses, dementia has also been described.[8] Parkinson's disease is treated by pharmacotherapy including anticholinergic medications, preparations of L-dopa (a dopamine agonist), and amantadine hydrochloride which stimulates the release of dopamine from the remaining intact dopaminergic neurons. Dopamine receptor agonists such as Parlodel (bromocriptine HCl), MAO inhibitors, and, occasionally, neuroleptic drugs are prescribed. These drugs have potential effects on mood, cognition, and perception. Surgical treatments have been used in some settings to decrease the symptoms of Parkinson's disease. These include lesioning specific areas of the brain, and tissue implantation into the striatum.[8] Other neurological diseases mimic the symptoms of Parkinson's disease, but their description is beyond the scope of this chapter.

Vocal tremor may have a variety of etiologies, and it is important to rule out serious causes such as cerebellar disease, Parkinson's disease, thyrotoxicosis, drug effects, and other causes. The most common cause of vocal tremor is essential tremor, also known as benign familial tremor. It is frequently associated with tremor elsewhere in the body, chiefly the head and neck, but it may involve only the voice. Tremor resulting from extremes of affect may need to be ruled out, and the psychological professional on the voice treatment team is charged with making this differential diagnosis. Voice therapy techniques are designed to maximize the patient's communication abilities by maximizing respiratory function, resonance, and articulation. Some patients also will benefit from pharmacological treatment.[6,8] In addition, the patient may benefit from short-term psychotherapy to address body image concerns related to the presence of the tremor and its effect on appearance and communication.

Stuttering also is associated with both neurologic and psychogenic etiologies and must be carefully differentiated by the laryngologist, neurologist, and speech-language pathologist before instituting interdisciplinary treatment.[10] Multiple areas of the nervous system are involved in the mechanism of stuttering. Developmental stuttering is very common in early life and usually resolves with maturation of the nervous system during the normal process of language acquisition. Stuttering is not common among professional voice users, and it is extremely rare for stuttering to affect the singing voice. Speech-language pathologists should be consulted for their expertise in the assessment and treatment of stuttering. The psychological professional ordinarily will treat stutterers on referral from speech-language pathologists and, occasionally, pediatricians. Interventions should be designed to enhance stress management, teach relaxation techniques, and address mood disorders and self-image concerns resulting from this communication pattern. There also is a form of stuttering due to brain injury, known as neurogenic stuttering.[10] This is seen most often in adults, and short-term psychological therapy is often appropriate adjunctively.

Myasthenia gravis is an autoimmune disease of the myoneural junction. Acetylcholine ordinarily depolarizes the endplate of a muscle fiber causing excitation and muscle contraction. In myasthenia gravis, the muscle fails to depolarize because of abnormalities involving the neurotransmitter acetylcholine. Myasthenia gravis occurs most commonly in women in their twenties and thirties and in men in their fifties and sixties. Muscles of swallowing and respiration, the ocular muscles, and the limbs are involved most commonly; but almost any area of the body may be affected. Myasthenia gravis also may be isolated to the larynx. In professional voice users, voice dysfunction may be the first symptom noticed by the patient.[6,8,9,11] The physician considers myasthenia gravis in a differential diagnosis whenever patients complain of voice fatigue, especially when it is accompanied by weakness or fatigue elsewhere in the body. Strobovideolaryngoscopic findings have been described by Sataloff.[6]

Laboratory testing (antistriatal muscle antibody and anti-acetylcholine receptor antibody), imaging studies (especially for thymoma), and electromyography with repetitive stimulation testing are used to establish the diagnosis. Tensilon is a drug administered intravenously to patients with presumed myasthenia gravis, after which they are observed for improvement of vocal quality and other symptoms. Drug therapy regimens for myasthenia gravis are designed to inhibit acetyl-cholinesterase or provide immune suppression. Some patients require surgical removal of the thymus gland; and if the disease cannot be adequately controlled medically, this may be recommended even though it puts the recurrent laryngeal nerves at risk. Plasmapheresis eliminates circulating antibodies and provides symptomatic relief. The speech-language pathologist will offer interventions to decrease the dysphonia and dysarthria and improve speech intelligibility and vocal endurance. The psychotherapist's contributions to the care of these patients address the issues that are inherent to the diagnosis of a chronic, progressive, life-altering disease.

Amyotrophic lateral sclerosis (ALS) is a degenerative, progressive, and fatal disease involving motor neurons of the cortex, brain stem, and spinal cord.[8,9] The etiology is unknown. Mean onset age is 56 years, and the disease is twice as common in men as in women.[8] Vogel and Carter report that in 50% of all cases, death occurs within 3 years after identification of the symptoms; approximately 10% of the patients survive up to 10 years, and some patients live as long as 20 years after diagnosis.[8] The entire body is eventually involved, and communication is impaired by a mixed spastic-flaccid dysarthria with severe compromise of speech intelligibility. A number of drugs have been tried in the treatment of ALS, but all have been disappointing. The initial therapeutic effects of the drugs eventually are overcome by the progression of the disease. Speech-language pathologists will treat these patients with interventions designed to improve communication and instruction in the use of augmentative communication devices as the disease progresses. Prostheses for palatal lift and surgical interventions using pharyngeal flaps have also been employed. The psychological professional's role in the care of these patients involves supportive counseling to the patient, family, and caregivers in the face of this fatal, tragic illness. Treatment of depression and family therapy interventions designed to refocus on the unimpaired cognitive and affective aspects of the patient will predominate.

Multiple sclerosis (MS) is a disease of the central nervous system that involves loss of myelin and lesions primarily in the cerebral cortex, brain stem, cerebellum, or spinal tracts. The diagnosis of MS is based on history and the diagnostic appearance of the brain on magnetic resonance imaging. Cerebrospinal fluid may demonstrate abnormal immunoglobulin production (oligoclonal bands) or myelin breakdown products. The disease is characterized by exacerbations and remissions. Five to 10 percent of patients develop a more chronic progressive illness.[8] The cause of multiple sclerosis is unknown, but it is clearly an autoimmune disease in which the helper T-cells attack and destroy myelin. Unfortunately, early in the disease progression when neurologic abnormalities are minimal many of these patients are diagnosed as anxious, depressed, hypochondriacal, or somatosizing. Both sensory and motor abnormalities appear as the disease progresses. Speech may eventually manifest a mixed flaccid, spastic, and/or ataxic dysarthria.

There is currently no known cure for multiple sclerosis, and drug therapy focuses on reducing the number of attacks or reducing the damage caused by each attack. Drug therapy is described in more detail in Chapter 5. Speech-language pathologists treat these patients to enhance intelligibility, and some patients may also undergo physical therapy for ataxia, tremor, and muscle weakness. Psychotherapy to address the associated depression, emotional lability, and occasional psychosis which may be the result of the disease or the drug therapy will be an integral part of these patients' treatments. Stress management, relaxation and imagery techniques, and general health-maintaining behaviors should be offered by psychological professionals with expertise in these areas.

Huntington's disease (Huntington's chorea) is an inherited disorder characterized by degeneration in the striatum (the caudate and putamen). The defective gene is carried on chromosome four. Onset is usually between the ages of 25 and 45 years, with an average duration of 15 years. Death usually occurs in the middle-fifties.[8] Symptoms include involuntary tics and twitching which gradually evolve into chorea with rapid, jerky, semi-purposeful movements, usually in the extremities. In the later stages, the movements become grotesque contortions, and dementia develops and progresses. The disease is diagnosed by history, genetic findings, and characteristic abnormalities of CT and MRI of the brain. There is no cure, and drug therapy is offered for the suppression of involuntary movement. The drugs themselves commonly cause extra-pyramidal symptoms and may also produce tardive dyskinesia. The psychological professional may become involved with these patients as they consider genetic counseling, advance directives, and opportunities to enhance interaction with significant people in their lives before the disease progresses to dementia. Supportive family therapy interventions also are required.

Gilles de la Tourette's syndrome is a dual neurological and psychiatric diagnosis. It is often familial, and onset may be as early as the first year of life. The median age at onset is 7 years. Tourette's syndrome is characterized by multiple motor tics and one or more vocal tics which worsen intermittently during the life of the affected individual. They tend to become more intense in periods of stress. Obsessive-compulsive behaviors may also coexist. Patients with Tourette's syndrome sometimes have dysphagia with incoordination of swallow. Vocal tics include involuntary sounds such as grunts, clicks, yelps, barks, sniffs, coughs, screams, snorts, and coprolalia (the uttering of obscenities) which is present in up to 50% of cases.[8,9,12] Drug therapy utilized in the treatment of Tourette's syndrome includes neuroleptics, clonidine, and pimozide. Psychotherapy is used to educate the patient and his or her family about the disorder. It often provides recognition of some characteristic features in other family members who may then be referred for medical treatment. Patients with Tourette's syndrome usually benefit from stress management techniques as emotional overload often increases the frequency and intensity of the tics. The psychotherapist often will be involved in urging compliance with drug therapy and will help to monitor and identify side effects.

Cerebrovascular accident (stroke) is a sudden, rapid onset of a focal neurologic deficit caused by cerebrovascular disease. Blood supply to the brain is disrupted, resulting in damage that affects the function of the part of the brain nourished by the damaged blood vessel. There are two primary mechanisms for a CVA: cerebral ischemia from cerebral thrombosis or cerebral embolism, or intracranial hemorrhage. Some patients experience strokelike symptoms which last for minutes or hours and then resolve. This is referred to as a transient ischemic attack (TIA). Strokes produce sudden loss of neurologic function including motor control, sensory perception, vision, language, visuo-spatial function, and memory.[8] CVAs cause a wide variety of communication difficulties including aphasia, dysarthria, and cognitive impairment. The features and extent of communication impairment depend on the site of lesion.

Treatment of CVA may include the use of thrombolytic agents to degrade clots, anticoagulants to prevent further clot formation, rehabilitative services including physical and occupational therapy, and speech-language therapy. Patients who have experienced CVA and their families require psychological support and care. This is ordinarily provided during the acute and rehabilitative phases of treatment. Neuropsychologists may perform formal testing, prescribe and implement cognitive rehabilitation, and offer psychotherapy for treatment of the affective consequences associated with such significant changes in level of function. Family therapy to support caregivers and significant others in the patient's life is often critical in allowing him or her to reestablish personal independence and the customary role within the family structure once rehabilitation is complete.

Spasmodic dysphonia is a term applied to patients "demonstrating specific voice sounds which may result from a variety of disease processes producing the same vocal result."[13(p499)] The etiology of spasmodic dysphonia has been attributed to organic pathology of the central and peripheral nervous systems.[9] Finitzo and Freeman reported that over 80% of their patients had associated central lesions with 50%

of them having a cortical lesion, primarily left perisylvian lacunar infarcts.[14] Spasmodic dysphonia may be *ADductor* or *ABductor* in nature. Vocal symptoms correlate with the type of dysphonia. Symptoms of adductor spasmodic dysphonia include strain, strangle, and intermittent voice breaks during vowels, consistently perceived as an effortful, harsh voice.[9] In abductor spasmodic dysphonia, the voice is normal or slightly strained, but interspersed with breathy spasms. In both types of spasmodic dysphonia, the onset is gradual. Mixed abductor and adductor spasmodic dysphonia also has been reported. Stemple et al note that spasmodic dysphonia is an insidious disorder and causes many psychosocial problems for those who display these symptoms. Many patients search for diagnosis and treatment for years and often may have seen numerous otolaryngologists, neurologists, psychologists, and speech-language pathologists before they receive definitive diagnosis.[5] Meige's syndrome (cranial dystonia) is a combination of oro-mandibular dystonia and blepharospasm accompanying spasmodic dysphonia. The respiratory muscles and those of the neck are variably affected.[15]

Every patient with symptoms of spasmodic dysphonia requires a comprehensive evaluation which should include laryngologic examination, strobovideolaryngoscopy, objective voice assessment, laryngeal electromyography, and evaluation by an experienced speech-language pathologist.[13] Most patients with spasmodic dysphonia have developed some compensatory muscular tension dysphonia which must be treated for the full extent of the spasmodic dysphonic component to be apparent. It is critical to make an accurate differential diagnosis between severe muscular tension dysphonia, psychogenic dysphonia (see Chapter 9), and spasmodic dysphonia before treatment is instituted. Serious systemic medical illnesses such as Wilson's disease may produce laryngeal dystonia and must be ruled out.

Once a diagnosis of spasmodic dysphonia has been made definitively, three basic treatment strategies are described in the literature: speech therapy, nerve destruction, and neuromuscular blockade. Therapy with an experienced speech-language pathologist will be critical in conjunction with any other therapy offered to these patients. Many patients will not manifest spasms during singing and may benefit from singing voice therapy which can then bridge into the use of the speaking voice. Neuromuscular blockade using Botulinum neurotoxin Type A (BoTox) is currently the most efficacious therapy available, although it is still considered "experimental" for this condition. The medication is injected into the appropriate intrinsic laryngeal muscle, generally under electromyographic guidance. The beneficial effect occurs over the 48 hours after injection. Side effects are usually transient and minor, involving breathiness and mild aspiration. The therapeutic benefit appears to persist for approximately 85 days.[13] Antibodies to Botulinum toxin may develop, but this is rare. Patients will benefit from continued therapy with a speech-language pathologist after Botulinum toxin injection to maximize vocal quality and efficiency.

The medical psychologist may participate in the diagnostic assessment of these patients, assisting in differential diagnosis. Identifying co-existing psychological issues and affective responses to the long and frustrating pursuit of accurate diagnosis and treatment is often beneficial in releasing bound-up psychic energy and helping the patient to return to a self-image congruent with the "healed" voice. This process is similar to that seen in patients who have undergone reconstructive plastic surgery and those who have accomplished significant weight loss. It is important to note that the "healed" voice is rarely fully restored to normal, and this realization may also require psychotherapeutic intervention.

Diseases affecting the cerebellum result in disorders of motor control. These may include hypotonia, weakness, fatiguability of muscles, and abnormalities in projected movement. A number of degenerative processes affect the cerebellum and its connections, but the one seen most frequently in adults is olivopontocerebellar atrophy (OPCA). This disease results in mixed ataxic and spastic dysarthria.[16] Disorders of cognition may also affect vocal communication. These include AIDS, Alzheimer's disease, and traumatic brain injury; but they are beyond the scope of this chapter. In all of these diseases, the medical psychologist's role is similar to that in other chronic, progressive degenerative disorders. The patient is assisted in maximizing identity and life contributions for as long as his or her physical, cognitive, and affective condition permits. Family members and significant others in the patient's life require support in order to continue to provide excellent quality, compassionate, respectful care and to retain and cherish their memories of the patient as he or she was prior to the onset and progression of the disease. Bereavement support also may be a component of care with this population.

The following case provides an example of the role of the psychotherapist in the care of a patient with a neurological condition affecting communication. She required diagnostic assessment by the medical psychologist to confirm the differential diagnosis of spasmodic dysphonia.

CASE EXAMPLE: SPASMODIC DYSPHONIA

This patient was a 50-year-old teacher in a public elementary school who used her voice to teach six classes daily, 5 days a week. She had no prior voice problems except for intermittent laryngitis approximately once yearly. For 18 months, she had been experiencing a sensation of strangulation with speech and a hoarse, raspy vocal quality during speech production. She had sought diagnosis and treatment 1 month after the onset of this symptom, and had already been evaluated by four otolaryngologists, one gastroenterologist, one allergist, and a speech pathologist. She related the onset of her vocal problems to the period immediately following a divorce and wondered aloud during her initial evaluation at the center whether she might still have some "unexpressed emotional reactions" to this event. Closely temporally related to the stress of the divorce was the potential for layoff from her employment. However, this had not happened. She had had no psychotherapy related to the divorce, work stress, or her vocal symptoms.

During her evaluation at the center by the speech-language pathologist and her examination by the laryngologist, she experienced episodes of clear voice during laughing, coughing, and immediately following swallowing. She also had short bursts of clear voice during her singing voice assessment.

To clarify the differential diagnosis between psychogenic dysphonia and spasmodic dysphonia, the patient was evaluated by the arts medicine psychologist. Self-report tools for stress and loss assessment, drawing assignments and a psychological interview were conducted. Four items of the life events and relative stress scale were rated as extremely negative, and they related to her divorce, potential layoff from her employment as a teacher, and the vocal illness itself. Her stress management strategies included painting, reading, exercise, and socializing with friends. She described as useful maintaining contact and discussing and listening to the counsel of significant others. She was in generally good health and usually attended to her needs for nutrition and rest. Her skills were well within the adequate range for time organization, relationship management, positive attitude, and physical self-care.

The grief inventory was also administered, and the patient endorsed a number of items in the affect domain, including sadness, shock, and anger which she described as her emotional reactions prior to diagnosis at our center. Emancipation and relief were also endorsed, and she described these as a direct consequence of receiving a clear medical diagnosis for her vocal difficulties. Behaviorally, she had been searching for diagnosis and cure and had been troubled by bouts of excessive crying. Cognitive distortions included a sense of disbelief, memory disturbance, and preoccupation with her "normal" voice. Physical sensations of tightness in the throat were consistent with her medical diagnosis.

Response to the art tasks included a realistic, representative self-portrait done in pencil and tinted with crayon. Interestingly, all color added to the picture was monotonal, and the patient's skin, hair, and lips were all done in a neutral beige hue. Facial asymmetry was noted, and the right side of the portrait revealed an eye with a direct, fixed gaze and a somewhat expressionless midface and mouth. The right side of the face included an upward and outward gaze as though fixed on something in the distance and increased muscle tone, as evidenced by lid position and facial lining. The mouth on the right side was also in the neutral position. There was significant shading under the chin and to the superior border of the larynx. The patient drew herself with a shortened neck.

Her drawing of her voice was an abstract representation of a model of the larynx. The tracheal rings were drawn in red at the level of the inferior glottis and progressed in slightly less intense hues through purple and pink. A soft, undefined, aqua area divided the trachea from the larynx itself. The thyroid cartilage was truncated into this dividing structure and was colored variously in hues of bright red, pink, and fiery orange. The same soft teal color appeared at the upper border of the larynx, spilling out in an active, almost "shotgun" style, and appearing in the lateral margins of the larynx. In the open area above the uppermost teal border were shapes drawn red and fushia. They were erratic and chaotic. Those in the uppermost section of the picture were softer in intensity and admixed with the color purple. The overall feeling of the picture was of a stable structure which was hot and intense, but was bisected by and floating in an oncoming ocean wave and producing and emitting energetic, but disorganized, matter.

The patient's psychological interview was completely within normal limits. Mental status showed no evidence of significant mood disturbance, anxiety, or thought disorder. Responses were verbally and nonverbally congruent. She had significant insight into the events surrounding her divorce and a prior marriage which also ended in divorce. She had been engaged in introspection about her relationship choices and the consequences. She described herself as assertive and communicated with evidence of knowledge and comfort with assertive communication techniques.

A preliminary relaxation exercise and hypnotic induction led to light trance with eyes open. The patient participated actively in an exercise allowing her to dissociate from a visual, auditory, and kinesthetic memory of herself in a situation of classroom stress when she remembered experiencing some frustration and aggressive thoughts toward children who were poorly behaved. She used her experience and professional skills to regain classroom order, but we explored her "desire to scream and rant" during imagery and allowed her to engage in her fantasy and observe the outcome. She was helped to identify markers for accumulating physical stress in the body, especially in the head and neck, and provided with cues and strategies for releasing the accumulating muscle tension and correcting the inhibitory respiratory pattern that accompanied it. The level of hypnosis was then deepened, and the patient was invited to communicate while in a profound state of muscle relaxation. The characteristic strain/strangled voice was still intermittently present during her verbal communications, even at a slowed rate of respiration and speech and profound muscle relaxation. The patient was assisted to emerge from trance, and strategies for general relaxation and improved emotional caretaking were described and discussed.

In consultation with the voice team, the arts medicine psychologist was able to assist the patient to address and remove the compensatory psychological patterns in much the same way that the speech-language pathologist and singing voice specialist had addressed and removed the compensatory muscle tension dysphonia patterns which had made the initial diagnosis of spasmodic dysphonia presumptive.

The patient received bilateral injections of Botulinum toxin and was reinterviewed 48 hours later. Her mood and level of physical and psychic energy had increased enormously. The voice was slightly breathy, but free of the qualities of strain and strangle. No hesitations were noted during the subsequent 1½-hour interview. During that session, the patient was assisted to use the Gestalt strategy of enactment with an empty chair to express her anger and disappointment at the prior care-providers who had not been able to make a definitive diagnosis of spasmodic dysphonia. She was also provided with current, updated information about the diagnosis of spasmodic dysphonia including the difficulty in assessment that sometimes delays definitive diagnosis. She continued to work with a speech-language pathologist and singing voice specialist to enhance her vocal effectiveness and to solidify her vocal hygiene habits as she returned to the classroom. The patient and the medical psychologist elected to schedule further psychotherapeutic interventions on an as-needed basis.

REFERENCES

1. Metcalfe R, Firth D, Pollack S, et al. Psychiatric morbidity and illness behavior in female neurological inpatients. *J Neurol Neurosurg Psychiatry.* 1988;51:1387-1390.
2. Gianotti G. Emotional behavior and hemispheric site of lesion. *Cortex.* 1972;8:41-55.

3. Alexander M, Loverme S. Aphasia after left hemispheric intracranial hemorrhage. *Neurology.* 1980;30:1193-1202.
4. Aronson A. *Clinical Voice Disorders: An Interdisciplinary Approach.* New York, NY: Brian C. Decker; 1980:71-115.
5. Stemple J, Glaze L, Gerdeman B. *Clinical Voice Pathology: Theory and Management,* 2nd ed. San Diego, Calif: Singular Publishing Group Inc; 1995;229-251.
6. Sataloff RT, Mandel S, Rosen, DC. Neurological disorders affecting the voice. In: Sataloff RT, ed. *Professional Voice: The Science and Art of Clinical Care,* 2nd ed. San Diego, Calif: Singular Publishing Group Inc; 1997:479-498.
7. Benninger MS, Crumbly RL, Ford CN, Gould WJ, Hanson DG, Ossof RH, Sataloff RT. Evaluation and treatment of the unilateral and paralyzed vocal fold. *Otolaryngol Head Neck Surg.* 1994;111(4):497-508.
8. Vogel D, Carter J. *The Effects of Drugs on Communication Disorders.* San Diego, Calif: Singular Publishing Group Inc; 1995:30-90.
9. Andrews M. *Manual of Voice Treatment: Pediatrics Through Geriatrics.* San Diego, Calif: Singular Publishing Group Inc; 1995:268-270.
10. Mahr G, Leith W. Psychogenic stuttering of adult onset. *J Speech Hear Res.* 1992;35:283-286.
11. Younger D, Lange D, Lovelace R, Blitzer A. Neuromuscular disorders of the Larynx. In: Blitzer A, Brin M, Sasaki C, Fahn S, Harris K, eds. *Neurologic Diseases of the Larynx.* New York, NY: Thieme Medical Publishers Inc; 1992:240-247.
12. American Psychiatric Association. *Diagnostic Statistical Manual of Mental Disorders—IV.* Washington, DC: American Psychiatric Association; 1994;71-73.
13. Deems D, Sataloff RT. Spasmodic dysphonia. In: Sataloff RT. *Professional Voice: The Science and Art of Clinical Care,* 2nd ed. San Diego, Calif: Singular Publishing Group Inc; 1997:499-505.
14. Finitzo T, Freeman F. Spasmodic dysphonia, whether and where: results of seven years of research. *J Speech and Hear Res.* 1989;32:541-555.
15. Richardson, Jr. EP, Flint Beal M, Martin J. Degenerative diseases of the nervous system. In: Braunwald E, Isselbacher KJ, Petersdorf RG, Wilson JD, Martin JB, Fauci AS, eds. *Harrison's Principles of Internal Medicine,* 11th ed. New York, NY: McGraw-Hill Book Company; 1987:2020-2021.
16. Gilman S, Kluin K. Speech disorders in cerebellar degeneration studied with positron emission tomography. In: Blitzer A, Brin M, Sasaki C, Fahn S, Harris K, eds. *Neurologic Diseases of the Larynx.* New York, NY: Thieme Medical Publishers Inc; 1992:279.

CHAPTER

13

Response to Vocal Tract Cancer

Everyone is susceptible to the development of laryngeal cancer; and it may occur at any age, although the incidence of laryngeal cancer increases markedly after the age of 50. In 1994, the American Cancer Society reported an estimated 12,500 new cases of laryngeal cancer (9800 for males, and 2700 for females) in the United States. The estimated total number of deaths from laryngeal cancer in 1994 is 3800.[1] The major etiologic factor is exposure to tobacco, and this is dose-dependent. Laryngeal cancer in nonsmokers is rare. Heavy alcohol use is also a factor and appears to work synergistically with tobacco, especially in the development of supraglottic tumors.[2] Additional risk factors include prior irradiation of the head and neck, inhaled pollutants, and leukoplakia or erythroplakia of the vocal folds.[3] Spiegel[4(p307)] notes that, because of the larynx's unique functions of voice and airway protection, treatment of laryngeal cancer has always been complex and controversial. Carcinoma of the larynx is known to be a potentially curable disease with an overall 5-year survival rate of over 67%, with early, smaller lesions offering a better opportunity for both survival and preservation of laryngeal function.[4(p307)]

Hoarseness is one of the seven warning signals of possible cancer listed by the American Cancer Society in all of its publications. Persistent hoarseness may motivate patients to seek medical examination because of fear of throat cancer. Early recognition of the symptoms of laryngeal cancer is critical to successful treatment. However, fear of cancer may cause otherwise rational individuals to react with denial and ignore symptoms until the condition becomes much more serious. Although denial can often be a successful and adaptive coping strategy for cancer patients during their treatment, it can also have negative consequences. Denial may reduce immediate distress at the diagnosis, but it may also have an extremely detrimental long-term effect, causing a patient to ignore symptoms and/or refuse evaluation and treatment. Professional voice users, because of the intimate relationship between voice and self, and voice and career, may delay seeking medical evaluation or may reject the necessary medical or surgical treatment.

Accurate assessment and staging (Table 13–1) is critical in determining treatment. Examination initially will be performed by fiberoptic laryngoscopy with video documentation. Stroboscopy is invaluable in determining the need for biopsy and the extent of tumor spread, especially in professional voice users.[4(p317)] Imaging studies, including CT scan with contrast infusion and sometimes adjunctive MRI scanning will be ordered. The surgeon searches thoroughly for another primary tumor in the aerodigestive tract because the rate of additional lesions is reported to be as high as 15%–30%.[5] The differential diagnosis of small glottic lesions includes hyperkeratosis, dysplasia, carcinoma in-situ, and invasive carcinoma. Pathologic tissue diagnosis is critical. After thorough evaluation and diagnostic biopsy, the surgeon will recommend treatment consisting of either surgery, radiation therapy, chemotherapy, or a combination of these modalities based on the patient's individual history, the tumor characteristics, and the potential effects on laryngeal function. The paramount concern in all of these decisions is the patient's chance for long-term survival, which should not be compromised by attempts to preserve laryngeal function. All le-

---

TABLE 13–1. Staging of Primary Tumor in Laryngeal Cancer.

Glottis

T_1 — Tumor limited to vocal cord(s) (may involve anterior or posterior commissures) with normal mobility.

T_{1a} — Tumor limited to one vocal cord.

T_{1b} — Tumor involves both vocal cords.

T_2 — Tumor extends to supraglottis and/or subglottis and/or with impaired vocal cord mobility.

T_3 — Tumor limited to larynx with vocal cord fixation.

T_4 — Tumor invades through the thyroid cartilage and/or extends to other tissues beyond the larynx.

sions, except invasive carcinoma, are treated by simple excision without large margins, followed by close observation.[4(p317)] Invasive cancer will require total surgical excision with clean margins and/or radiation therapy.

For most T_1 and T_2 glottic tumors, long-term cure rates after surgery or radiation are reportedly equal; and the treatment decision is made by comparing the time, complications of radiation therapy, and expense to those of the surgery.[4(p317)] Clinicians have assumed that radiation would not alter vocal quality as much as surgical procedures. However, no long-term study to evaluate this finding has yet been completed; and long-term dysphonia causally related to radiation may be severe. When tumor staging permits and voice is a primary concern, radiation therapy has been considered the best choice for initial treatment because of the belief that voice preservation is better than with surgery and because treatment failures from radiation can then be followed by surgery, although the complications are somewhat higher in irradiated patients.[4(p317)]

Radiation therapy usually involves 25–30 treatments administered over 6–7 weeks. The radiation dose (in cGY) will be calculated by the radiation oncologist and the head and neck surgeon. Once the area is identified, it is mapped with dye on the surface of the skin. Radiation kills malignant cells and some of the normal surrounding tissue during the treatments. Radiation may also be used with surgery for advanced laryngeal cancer, either pre- or postoperatively according to the surgeon's preference. Patients experience various side effects as a result of radiation which may include dysphagia, decreased taste, skin irritation, tissue swelling and hardening, decreased salivary flow, nausea, and damage to the teeth. These side effects are cumulative during the treatment and gradually subside when treatment has concluded, although some may be permanent.[6] Laryngectomy is surgical removal of the larynx. This may be partial or total and may also be accompanied by a radical neck dissection in which the lymph nodes and other structures of the neck are removed. A patient who has had the larynx removed is referred to as a laryngectomee.

Rehabilitation of the patient with laryngeal cancer is usually multidisciplinary. The team will include the surgeon, nurse-specialist, speech-language pathologist, dietician, and psychological professional. When the surgery has been extensive, physical therapists, audiologists, and radiation oncologists may also be included in the treatment team. Patients who undergo total laryngectomy may also be visited by volunteers from the American Cancer Society or the International Association of Laryngectomees.

Patients usually undergo a period of psychological adjustment following any disfiguring, cancer-related surgery. Not only does the person have to adjust to life as a cancer patient, but he or she is left with a major handicap, dysphonia, or, in the case of total laryngectomy, total loss of normal voice. As in all patients with a cancer diagnosis, the initial response is likely to be shock and numbness associated with the diagnosis and surgery. The experience of cancer is stressful for both patients and their families. Changes in health care delivery have drastically reduced much of the rehabilitation, physical care, and teaching that formerly took place in the hospital. Laryngectomy stoma care, tracheal suction, and tube feedings must be managed at home by family members. The disease and its treatment are often associated with numerous physical symptoms, and cancer patients face a multiplicity of potential losses, including loss of usual lifestyle, loss of job, loss of sense of control and mastery, perceived loss of lovability, loss of self-esteem and independence.[7] The overriding fear for most patients is the prospect of dying from their cancer.

Emotional reactions are wide-ranging and include anger and depression which may in part be related to the availability of support, time since diagnosis, progression of the disease, type of treatment, and various underlying personality factors.[8] The laryngectomized individual must make major psychological and social adjustments related not only to the diagnosis of cancer, but also with a sudden disability: the loss of voice. With improvement in prognosis, research has begun to focus on the laryngectomee's quality of life. Individuals must adapt to changes in communication (esophageal speech with or without a voice prosthesis), environment (humidity, contaminants), occupation (lifting, safety concerns), recreation (avoidance of water activities), and sexuality. There is wide variability in the quality of pre- and postoperative psychological support reported by patients during each phase of care. This is a crucial role for the voice team's psychologist.[9-14]

Coping may be defined as "constantly changing cognitive and behavioral efforts to manage specific external and internal demands that are appraised as taxing or exceeding the resources of the person."[15(p137)] This definition of coping is particularly applicable to a discussion of psychotherapy in individuals diagnosed with cancer for two reasons. First, the word "manage" emphasizes that coping does not necessarily entail mastery of the stressor. Second, the definition emphasizes that coping can be a cognitive process which does not always involve manipulation of the environment or the stressor itself. Using this definition, palliative strategies may also constitute effective means of coping. The psychological professional on the voice team will facilitate the grieving process related to the diagnosis of cancer and its inherent implications for loss of personal and professional self-definition as the patient experienced it prior to the diagnosis. He or she will facilitate the expression of a full range of affective responses and support the family, as well as the patient, during normalization. It may be useful to introduce the use of cognitive strategies such as redefining the stressful situation and selectively redirecting attention.

Given what is known about the contributions of cigarette smoking and immoderate consumption of alcohol to the development of laryngeal cancer, the psychologist may need to address guilt. The performing community (excluding opera singers), especially those within the highest incidence age group, appear to use alcohol and smoke in a higher distribution than society as a whole. Alcohol is a drug that is often self-prescribed for severe performance anxiety. Both alcohol and tobacco are notorious as part of social behavior at cocktail parties, for example. The loneliness of being "on the road," compromised social function, poor eating habits, and general neglect of their bodies and their overall health plague performing artists of all levels of professional success.

In addition, many professional vocalists who have not achieved significant financial success may not have access to health insurance and may further delay seeking medical treatment unless they consider the presenting symptom to be very serious. When these external factors are present, a difficult challenge exists for the psychologist involved in providing emotional support to a patient who has received a recent diagnosis of laryngeal cancer. What is required is the appropriate expression of affect while still maintaining sufficiently clear cognitive capabilities to make rational, well-considered decisions about treatment options. In addition, these patients need support throughout the postoperative or intra-radiation period and physical and psychological techniques to manage the inevitable symptoms.

Finally, the long-term outcome for the voice is unknown. Patients with a diagnosis of cancer describe a "time-bomb" existing within their bodies which may activate at any time, producing a recurrence of the cancer. In professional voice users, the change in vocal quality in the posttreatment period requires enormous psychological and technique adjustments, and it also serves as a reminder of the "time-bomb" every time they speak. The psychological consequences of this confluence of the patient's profession, self-image, and cancer awareness may be profound. The long-term impact on the voice itself often cannot be predicted with certainty, and patients must prepare for significant impact on their private and career use of voice.

REFERENCES

1. *Cancer Facts and Figures*. Atlanta, Ga: American Cancer Society; 1994.
2. Flanders WD, Rothman KJ. Interaction of alcohol and tobacco in laryngeal cancer. *Am J Epidemiology*. 1982;115:371-379.
3. Andrews ML. *Manual of Voice Treatment: Pediatrics Through Geriatrics*. San Diego, Calif: Singular Publishing Group Inc; 1995:301.
4. Spiegel JR. Surgery for carcinoma of the larynx. In: Sataloff RT, Gould WJ, Spiegel JR, eds. *Voice Surgery*. St. Louis, Mo: Mosby Year-Book Inc; 1993.
5. Larsen JT, Adams GL, Fattah HA. Survival statistics for multiple primaries in head and neck cancer. *Otol HNS*. 1990;103:14-24.
6. Stemple JC, Glaze LE, Gerdeman BK. *Clinical Voice Pathology: Theory and Management*, 2 ed. San Diego, Calif: Singular Publishing Group Inc; 1995:272.
7. Silberfarb PM, Greer S. Psychological concomitants of cancer: clinical aspects. *Am J Psychotherapy*. 1982:36:470-478.
8. Matt DA, Sementilli ME, Burish TG. Denial as a strategy for coping with cancer. *J Mental Health Counseling*. 1988;10:136-144.
9. Berkowitz J, Lucente F. Counselling before laryngectomy. *Laryngoscope*. 1985;95:1332-1336.
10. Gardner W. Adjustment problems of laryngectomized women. *Arch Otolaryngol*. 1966;83:57-68.
11. Stam H, Koopmans J, Mathieson C. The psychological impact of a laryngectomy: a comprehensive assessment. *J Psychosoc Oncol*. 1991;9:37-58.
12. New York City Committee. *Essentials of Cancer Nursing*. New York, NY: American Cancer Society; 1971:49-85.
13. Keith R, Shane H, Coates H, Devine K. *Looking Forward—A Guidebook for the Laryngectomee*. Rochester, MN: Mayo Foundation; 1977:1-43.
14. Sigler B, Schuring L. *Ear, Nose and Throat Disorders*. St. Louis, Mo: Mosby Year- Book, Inc.; 1993:171-259.
15. Lazarus RS, Folkman S. *Stress Appraisal in Coping*. New York, NY: Springer-Verlag; 1984:137.

CHAPTER

14

Stress Management

Stress pervades virtually all professions in today's fast-moving society. Whether one is a graduate student writing a dissertation, a singer preparing for a series of concerts, a teacher preparing for presentation of lectures, a lawyer anticipating a major trial, a businessperson negotiating an important contract, or a member of any other goal-oriented profession, each of us must deal with a myriad of demands on his or her time and talents. In 1971, Brodnitz reported on 2286 cases of all forms of voice disorders and classified 80% of the disorders as attributable to voice abuse or psychogenic factors resulting in vocal dysfunction.[1] However, regardless of its incidence, it is clear that stress-related problems are important and common in professional voice users. Stress may be physical or psychological, and it often involves a combination of both. Either may interfere with performance. This represents a special problem for singers, because physiologic manifestations of stress may interfere with the delicate mechanisms of voice production.

Stress is recognized as a factor in illness and disease and is probably implicated in almost every type of human problem. It is estimated that 50%–70% of all physician visits involve complaints of stress-related illness.[2] Stress is a psychological experience that has physiologic consequences. A brief review of some terminology may be useful. *Stress* is a global term that is used broadly. One common definition is the set of emotional, cognitive, and physiological reactions to psychological demands and challenges. The term *stress-level* reflects the degree of stress experienced. Stress is not an all or none phenomenon. The psychological effects of stress range from positive (eustress) to severely incapacitating (distress). The term *stress-response* refers to the physiological reaction of an organism to stress. A *stressor* is an external stimulus, internal thought, perception, image or emotion that creates stress.[3]

Two other concepts are important in a contemporary discussion of stress: *coping* and *adaptation*. Lazarus has defined *coping* as "the process of managing demands (external or internal) that are appraised as taxing or exceeding the resources of the person."[4(p283)] Lazarus and Folkman have also suggested that an individual's coping ability may influence tolerance for various forms of stress and divided ways of coping into two categories: problem-focused and emotion-focused. Problem-focused coping involves efforts designed to alter or manage the source of a problem; emotion-focused coping consists of efforts directed at reducing or managing emotional distress.[4]

In the early 1930s, Hans Selye, an endocrinologist, discovered a generalized response to stressors in research animals. He described their responses using the term *General Adaptation Syndrome*. Selye postulated that the physiology of the animals was attempting to adapt to the challenges of noxious stimuli.[3] The process of adaptation to chronic and severe stressors was physically harmful over time. There were three phases to the observed response: alarm, adaption, and exhaustion. These phases were named for physiologic responses described by a sequence of events. The *alarm* phase is the characteristic fight or flight response. If the stressor continued, the animal appeared to adapt. In the *adaptation* phase, the physiologic responses were less extreme but the animal eventually became more exhausted. In the *exhaustion* phase, the animal's adaptation energy was spent; physical symptoms occurred, and some animals died.[3]

Stress responses occur because mental processes in the brain via the limbic system and its interaction with the hypothalamus affect the entire body. A stressor triggers these brain centers which in turn affect target organs through nerve and endocrine connections. The brain has two primary mechanisms for the stress response, neuronal and hormonal, and these mechanisms overlap. The body initiates a stress response through one of three pathways: sympathetic nervous system efferents which terminate on target organs such as the heart and blood vessels; the release of epinephrine and norepinephrine from the adrenal medulla; and the release of various other catecholamines.[3] The sympathetic division of the autonomic nervous system is the arousal system. The stressor might be either external or an internal perception. The sequence of the events is as follows: A memory-image-thought is interpreted as danger, and the cortex of the brain responds. Next, the cerebral cortex, through various pathways, sends signals to the limbic system which adds emotional tone to the experience. The limbic system transmits impulses to the hypothalamus which regulates the autonomic nervous system, and the hypothalamus initiates a stress response in three ways. It sends signals to the anterior and posterior lobes of the pituitary gland which influences hormonal regulation throughout the body. It sends impulses to the adrenal medullae, initiating the release of epinephrine and norepinephrine, and it relays information to the pons which regulates such processes as heart rate, respiratory rate, and temperature regulation. From the brain stem, signals are relayed to the rest of the body via the sympathetic nervous system. The hypothalamus is the mediator between the cerebral cortex and the lower centers of the brain, and a link between the brain and the endocrine (hormonal) system. The hypothalamus also stores neuropeptides called enkephalins and may trigger the release of endorphins stored the pituitary, both of which are involved in pain control.

Recent, although contradictory, evidence indicates that the hypothalamus also can affect the immune system. The anterior lobe of the pituitary gland releases adrenocorticotropic hormone (ACTH) which travels through the bloodstream to the adrenal cortex. The posterior lobe of the pituitary gland releases antidiuretic hormone (ADH) causing the kidneys to retain water, thereby increasing blood volume and blood pressure. ADH, which is also called vasopressin, participates in the constriction of arterioles, another mechanism for raising blood pressure. The adrenal cortex releases two types of corticosteroids into the bloodstream, mineralocorticoids and glucocorticoids. Mineralocorticoids influence electrolyte balance, chiefly sodium and potassium. Aldosterone is a primary mineralocorticoid which causes the kidneys to retain sodium and water and increases blood volume and blood pressure. The main glucocorticoid is cortisol which, in addition to increasing blood sugar, increases circulating lipids and protein metabolism and reduces inflammatory and immune system response. Chronic stress also may affect other hormones released by the pituitary, including growth hormone, thyroid stimulating hormone, and reproductive hormones.[3]

Stress has numerous physical consequences. Through the autonomic nervous system, it may alter oral and vocal fold secretions, heart rate, and gastric acid production. Under acute, anxiety-producing circumstances, such changes are to be expected. When frightened, a normal person's palms become cold and sweaty, the mouth becomes dry, heart rate increases, his or her pupils change size, and stomach acid secretions may increase. These phenomena are objective signs that may be observed by health care professionals, and their symptoms may be recognized by performers as dry mouth and voice fatigue, palpitations, and "heartburn." More severe, prolonged stress also is commonly associated with increased muscle tension throughout the body (but particularly in the head and neck), headaches, decreased ability to concentrate, and insomnia. Chronic fatigue is also a common symptom. These physiological alterations may lead not only to altered vocal quality, but also to physical pathology. Increased gastric acid secretion is associated with ulcers, as well as reflux laryngitis and arytenoid irritation. Other gastrointestinal manifestations such as colitis, irritable bowel syndrome, and dysphagia are also described. Chronic stress and tension may cause numerous pain syndromes although headaches, particularly migraines in vulnerable individuals, are most common. Stress is also associated with more serious physical problems such as myocardial infarction (heart attack), asthma, and depression of the immune system.[3,5,6] Thus, the constant pressure under which many performers live may be more than a modest inconvenience. Stress factors should be recognized, and appropriate modifications should be made to ameliorate them.

Stressors may be physical or psychological, and often involve a combination of both. Either may interfere with performance. There are several situations in which physical stress is common and important. Generalized fatigue is seen frequently in hard-working performers and other professionals, especially in the frantic few weeks preceding major performances and deadlines. To maintain normal mucosal secretions, a strong immune system to fight infection, and the ability of muscles to recover from heavy use, rest, proper nutrition, and hydration are required. When the body is deprived of these essentials, illness (such as upper respiratory infection), voice fatigue, hoarseness and other vocal dysfunctions may supervene.

Lack of physical conditioning undermines the power source of the voice and cardiovascular endurance. A person who becomes short of breath while climbing a flight of stairs hardly has the abdominal, respiratory, and cardiac endurance needed to sustain him or her optimally through the rigors of performance. The stress of attempting performance under such circumstances often results in voice dysfunction. This correctable deficiency may shorten a performer's career if not corrected.

"Over-singing" is a common physical stress in singers. As with running, swimming, or any other athletic activity that depends on sustained, coordinated muscle activity, singing requires conditioning to build up strength and endurance. Rest periods are also essential for muscle recovery. A singer who is accustomed to vocalizing for 1 or 2 hours a day stresses his or her physical voice-producing mechanism severely when he or she suddenly begins rehearsing for 14 hours daily immediately prior to performances.[5]

Medical treatment of stress depends on the specific circumstances. When the diagnosis is appropriate but poorly controlled anxiety, patients usually can be helped by assurance that their voice complaints are related to anxiety and not to any physical problem. Under ordinary circumstances, once a singer's mind is put to rest regarding the questions of nodules, vocal fold injury, or other serious problems, his or her training usually allows compensation for vocal manifestations of anxiety, especially when the vocal complaint is minor. Slight alterations in tonal quality or increased vocal fatigue are seen most frequently, and often are associated with lack of sleep, over-singing, and dehydration in connection with the stress-producing commitment. The singer or actor should be advised to modify these problems and to consult the voice teacher. Voice teachers should ensure that good vocal technique is being used under performance and rehearsal circumstances.[5] Frequently, young singers are not trained sufficiently in how and when to "mark." For example, many singers whistle to rest their voices, not realizing that vocal fold motion and potentially fatiguing vocal fold contact occur when whistling. Technical proficiency and a plan for voice conservation during rehearsals and performances is essential under these circumstances. A manageable stressful situation may become unmanageable if real physical vocal problems develop.

Several additional modalities may be helpful in selected circumstances. Relative voice rest (using the voice only when necessary) may be important not only to voice conservation but also to psychological relaxation. Under stressful circumstances, performers need as much peace and quiet as possible, not hectic socializing, parties with heavy voice use in noisy environments, and press appearances. The importance of adequate sleep and fluid intake cannot be overemphasized. Local therapy such as steam inhalation and neck muscle massage may be helpful for some people and certainly does no harm. The laryngologist may be very helpful for alleviating the singer's exogenous stress by conveying "doctor's orders" directly to theater management, especially when the performer has difficulty with assertiveness and fears the discomfort of having to personally confront an authority figure to violate his or her "show must go on" ethic.[5] A short phone call by the physician can be helpful at this time. Exploration of long-term consequences of such self-defeating behavior can be addressed later. Patients should not hesitate to ask their laryngologist to make such a call if he or she does not offer to do so.

When stress is chronic and incapacitating, more comprehensive measures are required. If the manifestations of psychological stress become so severe as to impair performance or necessitate the use of drugs to allow performance, psychotherapy is indicated. The application of the dynamics of health and wellness in psychotherapy revolves around two major issues with regard to stress: how to eliminate stress and how to cope with stressors and be stress-resistant when stress cannot be eliminated. The goals of psychotherapeutic approaches to stress-management include: (1) modifying external and internal stressors, (2) changing affective and cognitive reactions to stressors, (3) changing physiological reactions to stress, and (4) changing stress behaviors.

The concept of stress resistance is fairly global. There are a multiplicity of approaches to being stress-resistant. A psychoeducational model is customarily used. Initially, the psychotherapist will assist the patient in identifying and evaluating stressor characteristics. A variety of assessment tools are available for this purpose, and some of these are included in Chapter 16. Interventions designed to increase a sense of efficacy and personal control are designed. Perceived control over the stressor directly affects stress level, and it changes one's experience of the stressor. Laboratory and human research have determined this to be one of the most potent elements in the modulation of stress responses.

Kobasa's research revealed that individuals who are physically well in spite of stress have a particular constellation of personality characteristics which she labeled "hardy." Hardy people have a strong commitment to work, family, friends, religion, political or altruistic endeavors; view change as a challenge; and experience a sense of personal control over their lives. These three Cs, commitment, sense of control, and challenge, are the essential ingredients of psychological hardiness.[7]

The *will to meaning* refers to the universal human need for meaningful purpose in life and the courage to create meaning. Viktor Frankl has written that "he who has a why to live for can bear with almost any how."[8] Personal experience and research suggest what most people intuitively know: meaning in life promotes life. That is, a sense of coherence results from the belief that something in life is worth the commitment, and this can turn unhappy experiences into challenges.

Social support, both given and received, appears to strengthen one's inner resources. Zarski and colleagues performed research on daily hassles, the irritating and frustrating demands that bother people day to day. Daily hassles, rather than dramatic life events, were found to be strongly associated with psychological symptoms, as well as with somatic illness.[9] Adler's work refers to the special role of social interest in influencing the impact of stressful events. This is defined as an innate personality variable and a key factor in determining psychological adjustment. The person with social interest is more inclined to rely on others, exists as part of a larger social whole, and is willing to contribute to the betterment of mankind.[10]

Rosenbaum[11] studied individuals who demonstrated hardy and resilient responses and a transformational coping style. He coined the term "learned resourcefulness" by which he meant a learned repertoire of basic skills that people use to successfully regulate their lives and confront daily hassles. Rosenbaum's research led him to believe that learned resourcefulness is the foundation of self-regulation. His research revealed strengths in four basic areas: cognitive skills, problem-solving skills, delay of gratification skills, and self-efficacy.[11]

In stress management therapy, concrete exercises which impose time management are taught and practiced. Patients are urged to identify and expand their network of support as well. Psychological intervention requires evaluation of the patient's cognitive model. Cognitive restructuring exercises as well as classical behavioral conditioning responses are useful, practical tools which patients easily learn and utilize effectively with practice. Cognitive skills include the use of monitored perception, thought, and internal dialogue to regulate emotional and physiological responses. A variety of relaxation techniques are available and are ordinarily taught in the course of stress-management treatment. These include: progressive relaxation, hypnosis, autogenic training, imagery, and biofeedback training. Underlying all of these approaches is the premise that making conscious normally unconscious processes leads to control and self-efficacy. These interventions are described more fully in Chapter 16.

As with all medical conditions, the best treatment for stress in performers is prevention. Awareness of the conditions that lead to stress (and its potential adverse effect on voice production) often allows the patient to anticipate and avoid these problems. Stress is inevitable in performance and in life. Performers must learn to recognize it, compensate for it when necessary, and incorporate it into their singing as emotion and excitement—the "edge." Stress should be controlled, not pharmacologically eliminated. Used well, stress should be just one more tool of the singer's trade.

REFERENCES

1. Brodnitz F. Hormones and the human voice. *Bull NY Acad Med.* 1971;47: 183-191.
2. Everly GS. *A Clinical Guide to the Treatment of the Human Stress Response.* New York, NY: Plenum Press; 1989:40-43.
3. Green J, Shellenberger R. *The Dynamics of Health and Wellness. A Bio-Psycho-Social Approach.* Fort Worth, Tex: Holt, Rinehardt and Winston Inc; 1991:61-64, 92, 98-136.

4. Lazarus RS, Folkman S. *Stress Appraisal and Coping.* New York, NY: Springer-Verlag; 1984:283.
5. Sataloff RT. Stress, anxiety, and psychogenic dysphonia. In: *Professional Voice: The Science and Art of Clinical Care.* New York, NY: Raven Press; 1991:195-200.
6. Stroudmire A, ed. *Psychological Factors Affecting Medical Conditions.* Washington, DC: American Psychiatric Press Inc; 1995:187-192.
7. Kobasa S. Stressful events, personality, and health: an inquiry into hardiness. *J Personality Social Psychol.* 1979;37:1-11.
8. Frankl V. *Man's Search for Meaning.* New York, NY: Pocket Books; 1963:167.
9. Zarski J, Bubenzer D, West _. Social interests, stress, and the prediction of health status. J Counsel Devel. 1986;64:386-389.
10. Adler A. *Social Interest: A Challenge to Mankind.* New York, NY: Capricorn Books; 1964:227-228.
11. Rosenbaum M. Learned resourcefulness as a behavioral repertoire for the self-regulation of internal events: issues and speculations. In: Rosenbaum M, Franks CM, Jaffe Y, eds. *Perspectives on Behavioral Therapy in the 80s.* New York, NY: Springer-Verlag; 1983:190-193.

CHAPTER

15

Performance Anxiety

Psychological stress is intrinsic to vocal performance. For most people, sharing emotions is stressful even in the privacy of home, let alone under spotlights in front of a room full of people. During training, a singer or actor learns to recognize his or her customary anxiety about performing, to accept it as part of his or her instrument and to compensate for it. When psychological pressures becomes severe enough to impair or prohibit performance, careful treatment is required. Such occurrences usually are temporary and happen because of a particular situation such as short notice for a critically important performance, a recent family death, and so on. Chronic disabling psychological stress in the face of performance is a more serious problem.

Of 2212 professional classical musicians surveyed by the International Conference of Symphony and Opera Musicians (ISCOM), 24% reported a problem with performance anxiety, and 16% described it as severe.[1] In its most extreme forms, performance anxiety actually disrupts the skills of performers; in its milder form, it impairs their enjoyment of appearing in public.[2] Virtually all performers have experienced at least some symptoms of hyperarousal during their performance history and all fear their reemergence. Some fortunate people seem to bypass this type of trauma, exhibiting only mild symptoms of nervousness before performance which disappear the moment they walk on stage. In these individuals, personal physiology works consistently for instead of against them. The human nervous system functions exquisitely for the great majority of our needs, but in performance anxiety it may work against the performer in the very circumstances during which he or she wants most to do well. Human autonomic arousal continues to be under the sway of primal survival mechanisms which are the basic lines of defense against physical danger. They prepare the individual to fight or flee in response to the perception of threat. These responses are essential to our survival in situations of physical danger.[3] The dangers that threaten performers are not physical in nature, but the human nervous system cannot always differentiate between physical and psychological dangers, and therefore it produces physiological responses which are the same. When the physical symptoms associated with extreme arousal are enumerated, it is easy to understand why they can be major impediments to skilled performance and may even be disabling. They include rapid heart rate, dry mouth, sweating palms, palpitations, tremor, high blood pressure, restricted breathing, frequency of urination, and impaired memory.[2]

This process is cognitive. Beck and Emery describe the development of cognitive sets using an analogy to photography.[3(p151)] The individual scans the relevant environment and then determines which aspect, if any, on which to focus. Cognitive processing reduces the number of dimensions in a situation, sacrifices a great deal of information, and induces distortion into the "picture." Certain aspects of the situation are highlighted at the expense of others, the relative magnitudes and prominence of various features are distorted, and there is loss of perspective. In addition, they describe blurring and loss of important detail. These are the decisive influences on what the individual "sees." They describe how the cognitive set influences the picture that is perceived. The existing cognitive sets determine which aspects of the scene will be highlighted, which glossed over, and which excluded. The individual's first impressions of an event provide information that either reinforces or modifies the pre-existing cognitive set. The initial impression is critical because it determines whether the situation directly affects the patient's vital interests. It also sets the course of subsequent steps in conceptualization and the total response to a situation.[3(p151)] According to the cognitive model, at the same time the individual is evaluating the nature of the threat, he or she is also assessing internal resources for dealing with it, and their availability and effectiveness in deflecting potential damage. The balance between potential danger and available coping responses determines the nature and intensity of the patient's stress response. Two major behavioral systems are activated in response to the threat, either separately or together: those mediated by the sympathetic branch of the autonomic nervous system ("the fight or flight response") and those related to the parasympathetic branch ("the freeze or faint response").[3(p40-50)]

One major feature of performance anxiety is that the actual fear prior to entering the situation appears plausible. According to DSM-IV, performance anxiety meets the criteria for specific phobia. That is, it includes the following:[4] (pp203-205)

1. Marked and persistent fear that is excessive or unreasonable, cued by the presence or anticipation of a specific object or situation,
2. Exposure to the phobic stimulus almost invariably produces an immediate anxiety response,
3. The person recognizes that the fear is excessive or unreasonable,
4. The phobic situation is avoided or else endured with intense distress,
5. The distress or avoidance significantly interferes with the person's . . . occupational or academic functioning,
6. The duration is at least 6 months (if >18 years old),
7. The anxiety associated with the situation is not better explained by another mental disorder."

In performance anxiety, a complex web of factors may aggravate the patient's fears. These include the relative status of both performer and evaluator, the performer's skill, his or her confidence in the ability to perform adequately in a given "threatening situation," and the appraisal of the degree of threat (including the severity of potential damage to career and self-esteem). The individual's threshold of automatic defenses which undermine performance, and the rigidity of the rules relevant to the performance in question are also factored into the intensity of the response. Unfortunately, the experience of fear increases the likelihood of the undesirable consequences. A vicious cycle is created in which the anticipation of an absolute, extreme, irreversible outcome makes the performer more fearful of the effects and inhibited when entering the situation.[3(p151)] Negative evaluation by judges or audiences is the psychic common threat. The individual suffering from performance anxiety believes that he or she is being scrutinized and judged. Components under observation include fluency, artistry, self-assurance, and technique.

Although most fears tend to decline with continued exposure and expertise, Caine[2] notes that even highly skilled performers do not always experience lessening of performance anxiety over time. Indeed, she describes a dilemma for the expert performer for whom a potentially humiliating and frightening mistake is less and less tolerable. Nagle[5] notes that "nothing could be worse than not having the opportunity to perform, yet when considering the potentially devastating effects of performance anxiety for those performers who are affected, nothing is more threatening than having that opportunity . . . . Public performance implies that musicians not only show competence, but also go beyond a mundane reading of the score to deliver an artistic and expressive interpretation with technical security and virtuosity."[5(p493)]

A behavioral feedback loop becomes established. The act of performance becomes the stimulus perceived as a threat. In situations of danger, the individual's physiology primes him or her to become more alert and sensitive to all potential threats in the surrounding environment.[2] Anticipating mistakes increases arousal, which further enhances access to memories of mistakes and feelings of humiliation, which activates more fears and more arousal. This process is linked by catastrophic thoughts, physiologic manifestations of anxiety, and imagery. Unfortunately, the process is often initiated very early in a young performer's training.

Pruett's[6] work on prodigies describes concern for young musicians who choose "an anxiety reducing pattern of grandiosity and omnipotence as a response to risks to self-esteem."[6(p345)] Self-esteem may become anchored to the possession of certain external qualities such as musical talent and success instead of the authenticity of the child's self-perceptions. This causes an increasing dependency on external admiration and adulation. Unconscious issues underlying anxiety of exposure in public are probably identical for performers and nonperformers. However, when rank in the most important domains of a young person's life is determined almost exclusively by demonstration of skill and competition, the pressure is relentless. Pruett[6] points out that youngsters need assistance in maintaining respect for their whole self and not merely their musicianship. Preservation of self-esteem should be a prime goal in the education of young performers. He recommends that these children receive instruction from their teachers, parents, and psychological professionals to "think of the people in the audience not as enemies, but as supportive, expectant colleagues and friends. Critics, like umpires, are part of the game."[6(p348)]

A variety of psychotherapeutic treatment approaches to performance anxiety have been described in the literature. Several are described in detail in Chapter 16. The most effective are cognitive and behavioral strategies that assist performers in modifying levels of arousal to more optimal levels. Cognitive therapy addresses the essential mechanism sustaining performance anxiety: the cognitive set a performer brings to the performance situation. The autonomic nervous system is merely responding to the threat as it is perceived, and the intensity of the response correlates to the degree of threat generated by the sufferer's catastrophic expectations and negative self-talk. Cognitive restructuring techniques are extremely effective in producing the necessary adjustments. Monitoring internal self-dialogue is the first step in recognizing the dimension of the problem. These excessively self-critical attitudes enhance the probability of mistakes. Homework exercises designed to monitor critical thoughts are assigned. In the second step of cognitive treatment, adaptive, realistic self-statements are substituted.

Behaviorally based treatment approaches such as thought-stopping, paired relaxation responses, and "prescribing the symptom" are also utilized. Hypnosis is very efficacious, providing relaxation techniques and introducing positive, satisfying, and joyful imagery. Brief psychotherapeutic approaches produce effective outcomes, but proponents of a more psychodynamic approach argue that the underlying conflicts will resurface in some form of symptom substitution. Nagle[5] relates childhood experiences and their intrapsychic significance as having effects not on the presence or absence of stage fright, but on the severity of an individual's reaction to appearing in public. In her formulation, the experience of being on stage as the focus of attention provides the catalyst for the activation of repressed psychic events and feelings.[5]

Our clinical intervention always includes an exploration for secondary gain offered by disabling performance anxiety. The performer's unconscious fear must be addressed for these treatments to remain effective and to avoid eventual symptom substitution. Patients are asked, "What does this symptom accomplish for you?" The question may sound unsympathetic, and the patient may need to search deeply for an answer. This search requires significant courage. If the patient makes effective use of the treatment strategies, what might be expected of him or her? Where might success lead? Is he or she ready to go on to the next phase in a performance career, or does it remain safer to be immobilized? Which problem is honestly more terrifying: the symptom of performance anxiety or the possibility of success? What would be the consequences of resolving the immobilizing performance anxiety? The patient is asked to imagine a life in which the problem is no longer present. This exploration is often conducted using the relaxation and enhanced perception available in hypnosis. Most of these questions are painful to answer. For some performers, success beckons with one hand and signals caution with the other. Eloise Ristad[7] describes this with extraordinarily pragmatic wisdom: "The part of us that holds back knows that change involves challenges—losses as well as gains. Change always means dying a little; leaving behind something old and tattered and no longer useful to us even though comfortably familiar."[7(pp154-155)] A successful psychotherapeutic response to disabling performance anxiety requires a thorough explanation of the personal meaning of the symptom to the patient as well as an extensive and exciting repertoire of strategies for effecting personal change.

Case Example: Performance Anxiety

This problem can be best understood by discussing a case example. Identifying details are altered to protect the patient, but the general content provides a view of the multifactorial issues and treatment approaches required. Ms. "S" was referred by her laryngologist for treatment of disabling performance anxiety. This problem was volunteered to the physician during history-taking. She was also diagnosed with gastroesophageal reflux laryngitis and muscular tension dysphonia. The patient had had vocal fold surgery performed 7 years prior to her evaluation. She described herself as an "hysterical personality." She had received psychoanalytic psychotherapy on two prior occasions for extreme anxiety and depression. By the patient's account, that treatment had offered her significant insight into her inter- and intrapersonal conflicts and defense mechanisms. However, her anxiety was recurrent and appeared in all situations during which her performance was perceived to be or actually evaluated.

At the time she first sought treatment, she was a full-time graduate student in a doctoral program and on fellowship. Ms. S had always maintained another occupation while developing her vocal performance career. Her undergraduate training and performance had been in another discipline. She subsequently added vocal performance and studied and performed supporting operatic roles until her vocal fold surgery. During the recuperation period, she maintained full-time employment in a business that subsequently experienced severe financial hardship. At that time, she applied to graduate school and was offered a teaching fellowship. During her initial session, her stated goals were: "to succeed in voice performance or be finished with it; and then to teach and write in my graduate school field."

Ms. S is the oldest of three siblings. She describes both parents as "failed performers" and felt that their hopes and dreams were "projected" on her. According to the patient, her "voice has always been my barometer," and her childhood illnesses all presented with throat symptoms and frequent loss of her speaking voice. At the time of her treatment, she had been married for 5 years. The marriage was being impacted by her anxiety, limited financial means, and decisions about achieving pregnancy.

Ms. S had sung "for fun" while traveling abroad on a sabbatical the prior year. She found herself surprised and delighted by the quality and agility of her singing voice and received acclaim from some European teachers. On her return, she resumed her vocal studies to the extent her financial situation permitted. She noted insightfully, "The better I get, the more overcome by anxiety I become. My technique shifts, and my tongue is full of tension." She voiced the awareness that she was, "so terrified by the idea of success that I shut myself down." She was unable even to vocalize alone because of overwhelming fears of doing harm to herself vocally. This had been present ever since her prior surgery. She described her voice as "free, attractive, and growing again" during her singing lessons. Under the watchful eye and tutelage of her teacher, she could experience relaxation and consistency. She felt that she was able to give her best performances in the studio because she felt "entirely dependent."

Ms. S was aware that she continued to be extremely cautious and protective about her vocal instrument. On the one hand, she feared doing it harm so that there could be no hope of a career as a professional singer. For example, one of the concerns she voiced about achieving pregnancy was of "vocal fold edema and permanent voice change." She also expressed concern about the timing of a pregnancy and care of an infant on upcoming performance opportunities. On the other hand, freedom from the looming demands of both success and failure as a performer were counter-balanced by equal tension toward other sources of acclaim, academic and marital.

Ms. S had benefited from her prior psychoanalytic therapy. She possessed extraordinary insight into the dynamics of her behavior and her ongoing conflicts. However, this awareness was not curative. Although she could identify and articulate transferential interactions in the therapy and in her external world, she could neither avoid nor interrupt them. A cognitive and behavioral approach to treatment was therefore selected. Psychoeducational approaches to the impact of cognition on behavior, as well as a thorough explanation of the physiologic responses to perceived threat were undertaken. Ms. S rapidly became adept at observing and identifying antecedent thoughts and their affective and physiologic outcomes. Initially, all assignments *avoided* the musical context. She was asked merely to observe and understand how her habitual cognitive set produced distressing affect and physical correlates in her body in many common situations. These were then extended to observations in her academic milieu and to her interactions with her husband.

The technique of restraining change was used until the patient was actively requesting permission to apply these assessments during singing lessons. The therapist continued to suggest that it would be premature to do so, and paradoxically, the patient began to engage in this form of self-analysis, "owning her own level of readiness." As the patient reported that she had "defied" the therapist for several weeks and brought written documentation of her observations, the therapist suggested that it would be useful to have a margin of safety in that context.

Using the Neuro-linguistic Programming (NLP) technique of visual-kinesthetic dissociation,[8] the patient was asked to remember a recent situation in the singing studio and attend to vivid visual, auditory, kinesthetic, and olfactory/gustatory experiences in the situation. She was then invited to "float up out of her body and take a vantage point in the room which allowed her to observe herself, her teacher, and any other relevant features of the studio environment. From that safe vantage point as a detached, intellectual observer, she could then make even more precise observations about her behaviors and responses in a setting replete with the formerly disabling anxiety. This was extremely beneficial, and she was able to identify facial expressions, voice tone shifts, trigger words and phrases, internal dialogue, and very early kinesthetic experiences of tension in the body she was observing before her. Using this gathered information, she was invited to "float back into herself" in the imagery and change the troubling cues. That is, she could imagine (or request) a change in the visual, auditory, or kinesthetic behaviors of the teacher. She could also dispute the internal self-talk and utilize muscle relaxation strategies previously learned and practiced to replace early muscle tension before it could grow to disabling proportions. This patient also benefitted from instruction in a variety of relaxation techniques, and audiotapes were made of individualized inductions and a self-hypnosis script. Role-playing assertive responses in habitually difficult and self-defeating interactions was also part of the treatment plan.

Finally, a number of strategies were used to assist this patient to retrieve the freedom and joy of singing which had led her to it. She was asked to consider several questions: "Why do you love music? What part does music play in your life? What is your overall musical goal?" She was asked to consider how making music made her feel and the way it affected her, and also what opportunities her music-making provided that she could not otherwise experience. Answering this kind of query requires reaching intimately personal parts of one's being and deep reflection.

For this patient, music was a way to learn more, to perform publicly, and to play out her fantasies. She was asked to "float through time and space and visit some of your favorite memories and fantasies of music-making." Quickly and with great freedom in her body, she arrived at a memory of singing and dancing for her grandmother at approximately age 4. This grandmother was a person who gave her the gift of unconditional love and total affirmation. She was invited to apply those feelings of "floating within love and acclaim" to each and every experience which resonated with those feelings. They were auditorily and kinesthetically anchored during the session. This anchor was later overlapped with a visual icon of the patient's own creation. The anchors were then tested in imagery by inviting the patient to revisit scenes from her past in which her performance anxiety had been disabling and to fire the anchors, allowing a new resources to flood the old memories. They were then future-paced into upcoming auditions and future goals. Finally, the patient created in imagery a formerly phobic scene, at first dissociated and then "stepping into the picture" in an associated state, taking with her the new resources. Physiologic observations and the patient's self-report suggested that this was very successful and an emotionally prudent and moving experience for her. Ms. S terminated therapy, completed her doctoral studies, conceived a child, and continues to study and audition.

Knowledgeable psychotherapists design interventions for each patient based on individual assessment of the components contributing to the problem and the available coping resources. Performance anxiety is a critical problem for affected professional voice users. Efficacious treatment requires additional mastery of the physiological psychology of the stress response and empathic insight regarding performance demands.

REFERENCES

1. Fishbein M, Middlestadt S, Tattati Z, et al. Medical problems among IC-SOM musicians: overview of a national survey. *Med Prob Perf Art*. 1988;3:1-8.
2. Caine JB. Understanding and treating performance anxiety from a cognitive-behavior therapy perspective. *NATS*. 1991;27-51.
3. Beck A, Emery G. *Anxiety Disorders and Phobias: A Cognitive Perspective*. New York, NY: Basic Books Inc; 1985.
4. American Psychological Association. *Diagnostic and Statistical Manual*. Washington, DC: American Psychological Association; 1994:203-205.
5. Nagle JJ. Stage fright in musicians: a psychodynamic perspective. *Bull Menninger Clin*. 1993;4:492-503.
6. Pruett KD. Psychological aspects of the development of exceptional young performers and prodigies. In: Sataloff RT, Brandfonbrener A, Lederman R, eds. *Textbook of Performance Arts Medicine*. New York, NY: Raven Press; 1991:337-349.
7. Ristad E. *A Soprano on Her Head: Right Side Up Reflections on Life and Other Performances*. Moab, UT: Real People Press; 1982:154-155.
8. Lankton S. *Practical Magic: A Translation of Basic Neurolinquistic Programming into Clinical Therapy*. Cupertino, Calif: Meta Publications; 1980:110.

CHAPTER

16

Psychotherapeutic Management of the Voice-Disordered Patient

All mental health professionals specialize in attending to the emotional needs and problems of human beings. There are several different disciplines in which this expertise may be gained and credentialed. *Psychiatrists*, as physicians, focus on the neurological and biological causes of treatment of psychopathology. Consultation liaison psychiatry is the subspecialty of psychiatry that deals with the psychiatric problems of medical and surgical patients. Some psychiatrists are also psychoanalysts and utilize psychotherapy as a primary treatment modality. *Psychologists* have advanced graduate training and licensure in psychological function and therapy. They concern themselves with cognitive processes such as thinking, behavior, and memory; the experiencing and expression of emotions; significant inner conflicts, characteristic modes of defense in coping with stress; personality style and perception of self and others, including their expression and interpersonal behavior.

Licensed mental health counselors and *licensed clinical social workers* are also providers of psychotherapeutic services. Mental health counseling emphasizes "a focus on high level well-being, rather than simply the absence of disease," and "a holistic view of the client as a person consisting of interrelated domains of life."[1] In addition to training in the theory and practice of psychotherapy, licensed clinical social workers also receive advanced training in "development and application of a helping technology which deals with the problematic aspects of a person's role performance, whether caused by factors internal or external to the person. It is therefore not only concerned with change in the individual, but with change in the social environment when that environment is assessed as inimicable to the well-being of its members."[2(p1)] Psychiatric Nurse Clinical Specialists are Registered Nurses with graduate-level education in psychiatric disorders. They utilize nursing diagnosis to assess, plan, implement, and evaluate mental health care in inpatient and outpatient settings.

Consultation liaison psychiatrists, medical psychologists, and medical social workers specialize in the application of physiologic psychology, psychosomatic medicine, and altering the social and environmental maladaptations which are responses to illness or injury. Subspecialty training in any of these disciplines is often difficult to acquire. Although some graduate or postdoctoral training programs exist in each of these disciplines, gaining expertise after generalized training and credentialing often requires a personal search. A great deal of theoretical and clinical knowledge comes from scouring interdisciplinary literature, attending workshops and seminars, and designing mentorship, internship, or fellowship experiences with recognized experts in the field. Although interdisciplinary graduate programs have been proposed in the literature,[3] there is no academic program for the credentialing of arts-medicine psychologists. Therefore, the professional who wishes to work at a high level of clinical excellence, based on a sound knowledge of theoretical principles, must master information in the fields of psychology, medicine, speech-language pathology, audiology, ophthalmology, orthopedics, physical therapy, occupational therapy, vocal pedagogy, and music.

Psychological professionals working with performers may encounter them in a variety of practice settings, as well. Those with inpatient privileges may visit performers while they are hospitalized as a result of an injury or illness. The majority of psychological professionals will care for these patients on referral from a physician, speech-language pathologist, physical or occupational therapist, singing teacher, instrumental music teacher, or acting teacher. The importance of open communication with other professionals providing care for the performer cannot be overemphasized. The psychotherapist must be certain to clarify the limits of confidentiality with the patient immediately, so that sufficient information to offer well-tailored, appropriate intervention occurs without violating privilege. Perhaps the most rewarding setting for psychological intervention is an Arts Medicine Center where the psychological professional functions as a member of the treatment team, working directly with some patients and offering consultation to the physician and other professionals in designing and implementing care.

As has been previously described in this text, some patients are referred to the psychological professional for a formal psychological interview to clarify the differential diagnosis. Personality assessment, screening for or evaluating known psychopathology, and assessing many potential surgical candidates are also performed. Occasionally, psychometric instruments are added to the diagnostic interview. In this setting, confidentiality of content is extended to the entire treatment team so that interdisciplinary care is maximized. Occasionally, the psychological professional is present during the physician's history and physical examination and gathers information through observation during that process at the physician's request. Because of their special interest in voicing parameters, psychotherapists serving on voice treatment teams should be especially attuned to the therapeutic use of their own voices for intensifying rapport and pacing/leading of the patient's emotional state during interventions.[4-8]

Psychotherapeutic treatment is offered on a short-term, diagnosis-related basis in this setting. Treatment is designed to identify and alleviate emotional distress and to increase the individual's resources for adaptive functioning. Individual psychotherapeutic approaches include brief, insight-oriented therapies, cognitive/behavioral techniques, Gestalt interventions, stress management skill building, and clinical hypnosis. This text is not intended to offer psychological professionals adequate instruction to perform treatment interventions for which they have not received prior clinical credentialing. The author (DCR) has found the theories and techniques of neurolinguistic programming (NLP) and Ericksonian hypnosis particularly efficacious in this patient population. They are also enormously powerful and should not be applied by clinicians not trained to recognize contraindications and manage potential complications. Interested readers are referred to several comprehensive texts and training programs.[7-15]

After any indicated acute intervention is provided, and in patients whose coping repertoire is clearly adequate to the stressors, a psychoeducational model is used. The therapy session focuses on a prospective discussion of personal, inherent life stressors, physiologic responses to chronic and acute stress, and predictable illnesses. Stress management skills are taught, and audiotapes of the sessions are provided. These offer portable skills to the performer, and supplemental sessions may then be scheduled by mutual decision during appointments at the center for medical examinations and speech, singing voice, or acting voice therapy.

GROUP THERAPY

A group therapy model, with professional facilitation, has also been used to provide a forum for discussion of patient responses during the various phases of treatment. Participants benefit from the perspective and progress of other patients, the opportunity to decrease their experience of isolation, and the sharing of resources. A common reaction among these patients is that no one understands them well enough to be of assistance. Well meaning members of their support system or other professionals who have not "been there" have little credibility and are often rejected as sources of support. These patients often feel isolated because of the failed attempts by others to assist them. Family or friends may have offered platitudes, implied that the experience is trivial, said that they understand when it is obvious that they experientially cannot; or they have avoided the issues most important to the patient who perceives a potential or actual loss of voice.

Often patients then come to resent members of their natural support system for their failure to provide effective support, and they conclude that they are alone in their distress. According to Tedeschi and Calhoun,[16] many patients who have experienced recent loss seek help from those who have credibility and understanding derived from personal experience. They seek to avoid the negative, unhelpful responses of people who have not experienced the same trauma, to find people to whom disclosure of emotionally charged experiences and reactions will be less embarrassing, and they search for models of adjusting to the difficulties they face.

Carpenter[17] has described her experience with a voice support group which "provides a forum for individuals to discuss their experiences, share both their positive and negative feelings, and begin to gain control and rebuild the voice." Before surgery, patients use the group to discuss anxieties and fears and have an opportunity to hear others share their experiences. Following surgery, patients share their progress and frustrations with others who can empathize and encourage them. At follow-up, participants revealed that they felt better and more in control of their surgical experience, as well as experienced a lessening of fear and anxiety and a more positive attitude about the outcome of surgery.

Different issues are of concern at various points in the treatment process, and group members need different experiences with the group at different times. Initially, new group members find comfort in being accepted to this community of like persons, but admission to the group is also an admission of one's status as a voice-injured professional. However, attending the group for the first time is a step through the denial. As others recount their similar experiences, the stories often produce emotional reactions in group members and an implicit expectation of self-disclosure is sometimes difficult, especially for new members.

In the middle stages of the group, isolation is eased by the perception of similarity of experience in treatment. Especially valuable is recognition that the processes involved in coping are virtually universal and that revelations of potentially embarrassing topics are tolerated. Facilitators assist each patient in finding a subgroup of members with similar experiences, opinions, and coping methods. Veteran group members also are able to credibly challenge newer group members and those less successful with their coping attempts to experiment with other methods. In the later stages of group development, patients bring into the group the discovery that individuals exist outside the group community who have the potential to be good sources of support, and the group begins to lose some of its special quality and significance. This is a crucial development in setting the stage for group termination. This takes place as group members have begun to re-identify with the "normal" population and to use support available in their existing social world.

The usual challenges to the credibility of the therapist are certainly demonstrated, and the psychological professional facilitating such a group is better accepted if he or she shares at least some aspect of group identity, usually the performer role or the patient role. We have experimented with conducting these groups using both open- and closed-ended models. Each has its advantages and disadvantages, and they are not dissimilar from those found in the literature on group processes in general. Where co-therapists are involved, both professionals must be willing to use peer or mentor supervision when interpersonal issues threaten to impede group work. This is, of course, an ethical obligation for therapists working in any setting.

Long-term psychodynamic psychotherapy, chronic psychiatric conditions, and patients requiring psychopharmacologic management are referred to consultant psychotherapists and psychiatrists with special interest and insight in performance-related psychological problems. The voice team's psychologists also serve a liaison role when patients already in treatment come to the voice center for care. In this setting, the psychological professional's mandate is for short-term, treatment-related emotional distress. Longer term therapy directed to personality change or for the reinforcement of new cognitive or behavioral strategies is best managed by colleagues in the community. The initiation of drug therapy or the modification of existing therapy where drug side effects play a significant role in the vocal problem are handled by direct communication between the laryngologist, voice team psychological professional, and the psychiatrist. Psychophysiological research informs our treatment and maximizes benefits to patients in every specialty. In addition to direct care, the arts medicine psychologists at the voice center participate in professional education activities. These include writing, lecturing, and serving as a preceptor for visiting professionals.

FAMILY THERAPY

Significant vocal impairment affects human communication and body image. This impacts not only on the patient with the injury, but also the family, whether traditionally or nontraditionally defined. Walsh and McGoldrick note that the family approaches and reacts to loss as a relationship system, with all members participating in mutually reinforcing reactions.[18] According to their research, loss has implications for how the family will adapt to later experiences, as patterns set in motion because of significant loss for any family member have both immediate impact and long-term ramifications in family development, potentially across several generations. Reaction to loss is one of the normative transitions in the family life cycle; and as such, carries the potential for growth and development, as well as distress and long-term dysfunction. Families influence how the event is experienced. So, as the clinician attends to family processes, he or she can promote healthy adaptation to loss and strengthen the family unit in meeting other life challenges. When assessing families during therapy, it is critical to attend to the legacies of past losses in the family system, as well as to cultural diversity in the grieving process.[18]

INDIVIDUAL PSYCHOTHERAPY

However, the majority of psychotherapy is performed by the psychotherapist directly with the patient experiencing the medical illness. There are numerous models of the counseling process, and each practitioner will be influenced by his or her theoretical and clinical training. Health care economics in the 1990s has dictated the use of brief therapy models with measurable outcomes. These are certainly appropriate for psychological professionals functioning within the medical care team, but the basic elements of the counseling process are nevertheless maintained. In general, they consist of three phases: *the initial phase* in which rapport, contracting for change, and problem identification occur; *the middle phase* in which psychological issues that relate to the medical problem are explored further and clarified, allowing the patient insight into the psychological determinants of the symptoms and the generation of alternative responses; and *the final phase* in which these interventions are delivered, practiced in the patient's external world, and refined. This is also the phase of termination which offers patients the experience of a more adaptive method of responding to a necessary loss.

It is a truism of all psychotherapy that the therapist is merely a well educated guide who makes accurate, informed assumptions about the areas in which the origin and maintenance of psychological distress dwell. However, the patient does the work of healing alone. At some point in their training, all therapists learn to be attentive to situations in which they are working far harder than the patient, because "ownership" of the problem and investment in its outcome are critical to success, regardless of the counseling model. Shakespeare, with customary brilliance, reminds us of this in MacBeth as MacBeth discusses the deteriorating mental health of his wife with her physician:

> Canst thou not minister to a mind diseas'd,
> Pluck from the memory of rooted sorrow,
> Raise out the written troubles of the brain,
> and with some sweet, oblivious antidote
> cleanse the stuff'd bosom of that perilous stuff
> which weighs upon the heart?

And the physician replies:

> Therein the patient
> must minister to himself.[19(p1052)]

All therapy begins when the psychotherapist and the patient create a positive alliance in which rapport is established and the therapist offers accurate empathy and unconditional acceptance. Medical psychologists maintain a theoretical stance that some symptoms may reflect underlying psychological distress and that all symptoms, whatever the cause, have an emotional component. Furthermore, there is nothing abnormal in the patient's reaction of distress; it is a normal response to a painful experience. The goal is to establish the connection between symptoms, affect, and somatic distress. In some instances, a single interview in which the patient is able to develop conscious awareness of the interrelationship between his or her psychological needs and physical symptom may be sufficient. Patients continue to process profound insights which are achieved during a therapy session, and this working-through may be conscious or unconscious.[20]

All human beings possess a basic desire to heal and grow toward emotional maturity, even though there may be a powerful counterbalance of resistance. Resistance is here defined as a defense against emotional pain, the purpose of which is to prevent the return of repressed, distressing emotions to the patient's conscious awareness. At some level, most individuals will demonstrate a reluctance to give up psychological symptoms and the protection they provide. Changing existing emotional patterns requires acknowledgment that previous behavior has been inappropriate, and this may be especially deep-seated when behaviors and attitudes have become central to much of that person's life definition. Almost every psychotherapist has encountered individuals who fear that, if they change markedly, they will no longer recognize what they consider to be central to themselves.

A patient's need for symptoms and defenses must be explored and worked through before the physical and psychological advantages of possessing the symptom can be relinquished. Therapists must remember that the patient has consented to psychotherapy in order to become more aware of his or her problems and discover how to live and deal with these concerns in ways that fit appropriately in "real life." It is the therapist's goal that the patient will leave therapy capable of encountering future problems and dilemmas with more skills to understand and resolve them as a result of the therapeutic process and to discover methods for finding his or her own way alone through future problems.

It is a great error for therapists to attempt to strip patients of all defense mechanisms. In clinical practice, we must be very explicit about the benefit of holding on to defense mechanisms as valuable and effective in having allowed the patient to successfully negotiate and survive the dangers and vicissitudes of his or her personal life experiences. Patients are helped to examine defense mechanisms, become better acquainted with them, and "befriend" them. When the old defense mechanisms are no longer necessary, they are placed in an "honored place," able to be retrieved if necessary. Clinicians should convey great respect for the unconscious parts of self that are responsible for behaviors that are intended to protect, regardless of the maladaptive ways in which they are manifested.

In almost every case, when patients are seeking change, conflict exists between their conscious desires and some unconscious set of programs. Bandler and Grinder caution therapists to remember that the unconscious is far more powerful, knows more about the needs of the patient than the conscious mind, and is more accurate than the therapist.[10] One of the techniques used frequently in the authors' clinical practice when searching for secondary gain of distressing symptoms is the neurolinguistic programming (NLP) technique of *six-step reframing.* This process is described in detail in Chapter 9.

INITIAL PHASE OF THERAPY

During the initial phase of therapy, one of the clinician's tasks is to assess the patient's personality and his or her characteristic response to illness. This is one of the components of a psychological interview and will be helpful in predicting the interventions which may become necessary, because defensive styles of most people become temporarily magnified by the experience of illness. The patient's age and developmental stage will also be critical because the meaning of illness is clearly different at each stage of life. Medical psychologists must also understand and assess the nature of the disease or injury itself, including its rate of onset, degree of impact on interpersonal and occupational functioning, and likely medical course. This is one area where membership in a treatment team is invaluable. The clinician remains constantly observant of the impact of the physical problem on the patient's family and social support system, maintaining an awareness that affective ties to family and friends may be strengthened or disrupted, and memories of prior losses and illnesses revivified.

During the initial phase of the counseling relationship, a therapeutic contract will be developed. The change contract is simply a statement of what the patient intends to accomplish by entering the therapeutic relationship. Ron Klein suggests that the therapist ask the patient the simple question, "What do you want to do differently?" (Ron Klein, personal communication), after hearing a description of the current problem and observing the nonverbal and paraverbal responses in the problem state. A clear contract exists when the answers are: (1) stated positively; (2) measurable or verifiable by external means; (3) initiated and maintained by the patient; (4) within the patient's power to accomplish without changing the behaviors of others; and (5) "ecologically sound" in the patient's world of reality.[9]

How patients cope with the stress of illness depends to a large extent on the meaning of the illness to them, that is, on their *cognitive appraisal* of the situation. In addition to unconscious psychological defenses and psychodynamic interpretations, this involves an active, conscious problem-solving strategy, and it will have different manifestations during different phases of the illness.[21] Individuals should be assessed with regard to their personal beliefs, attributions, concepts, expectations, predictions, and the inner statements they make to themselves about life experiences.

The therapist will emphasize the importance of understanding the interrelation between cognitions (thoughts and imagery), emotions, physiologic reactions, behavior, interpersonal relationships, life events, and the escalation of symptoms through negative self-talk.[22] Assessment of the "ABCs," the *antecedent* event, the *beliefs*, and the *consequences,* is central to this theory. Understanding the patient's dysfunctional thinking is a mutual process in which both the patient and therapist are engaged. Patients are taught to complete daily "thought records" as a means of enhancing their skills and making the connection between these three components. Numerous forms are available and are described in detail by Beck and colleagues.[23,24]

Specific appraisal of coping styles is also conducted, and several models exist. Weisman divided coping responses into three categories: (1) appraisal-focused responses which involve logical analysis such as cognitive redefinition and cognitive avoidance; (2) problem-focused responses which involve more active information seeking, problem solving, or development of alternative rewards; and (3) emotion-focused responses which involve affective regulation, emotional discharge, and resigned acceptance.[25] Amatea and Fong-Beyette classified coping responses into nine types: six active and three passive. The active types of coping were described as increasing planful role behavior, internal role redefinition, external role redefinition, cognitive appraisal, tension reduction, and use of social support. The passive types of coping were reactive role behavior, rigid role definitions, and the use of intra-psychic defenses such as blame or wishful thinking.[26]

Dr. Nicholas Rosa (personal communication) cautioned his graduate students to remember that, in any psychotherapeutic encounter, both the patient and the therapist come with a repertoire of behaviors. For therapy to be effective, the therapist's repertoire must be the larger one. "He or she with the greatest repertoire wins." That is, for every problem and "Yes, but" response, the therapist must have the ability to reframe the inadequate response as an experiment offering data and have at least one more way to address the self-defeating response. Thus, we favor an eclectic clinical approach, combining effective strategies and techniques from every theoretical school of psychotherapy. Eclectic, however, is not equivalent to atheoretical. It merely means that every psychotherapeutic method is effective for some patients and for some psychological problems some of the time. In the remainder of this chapter, some of the author's (DCR) approaches to psychotherapy in voice-disordered patients are described. To enhance accessibility, they are described by the voice disorder they are being utilized to treat, organized in accordance with the topic headings in the previous chapters.

PSYCHOGENIC DYSPHONIA

The stage of rapport is especially critical in dealing with these patients because of the characteristic defenses around the symptoms themselves. In addition to the clinician's usual rapport building skills, the Neurolinguistic Programming (NLP) skills of pacing, sometimes known as mirroring, are particularly helpful in gaining rapport with clients and joining them in their model of the world. Bandler and Grinder coined these terms after modeling the communication behavior of particularly masterful communicators such as Milton H. Erickson and Virginia Satir.[10] They teach that to the extent the therapist can match another person's behavior, both verbally and nonverbally, the therapist will be pacing the patient's experience. Pacing is truly the essence of what most clinicians call rapport.

Two types of nonverbal pacing exist. One is *direct mirroring*, for example, breathing at the same rate and depth as the patient; and the other is *crossover mirroring*. This approach substitutes one nonverbal channel for another. In this method, the therapist may use subtle hand movements to pace the rate of rise and fall of the chest during breathing, or *pace* the rate of speech during hypnotic intervention to the rate and rhythm of the patient's breathing. Once the pace behaviors truly match the experience of the client, the therapist *leads* the patient into new behavior by changing what he or she is doing through *overlapping*. Nonverbal mirroring is a powerful unconscious mechanism used by all human beings who communicate effectively. Most clinical therapy tends to underemphasize the importance of sensory data available from the eyes, ears, skin, nose, and when people communicate.[7]

Each human being has available a number of different ways of representing the experience of the external world. These are called *representational systems*, sensory processing systems that initiate and modulate behavior. Some of the information received through sensory channels is conscious, and some is unconscious; but it is all translated by human beings into internal representations that eventually influence our behavior. Information is taken in through all sensory channels, processed through a few uniquely individual favored channels, and finally fed back to the external world through behavior in particular sensory modes. The primary representation system is the processing channel of which the person is most conscious.[7] Patients use predicates during communication which can alert the trained therapist to the sensory system the patient habitually prefers. This literally allows the therapist to be "speaking the patient's language."

Finally, practitioners of Neurolinguistic Programming and Ericksonian hypnosis are particularly attuned to eye accessing cues during communication. These should be initially calibrated for every individual using simple questions during which patients are asked to remember prior events. The therapist can then obtain information about the direction of eye movement utilized when the patient experiences remembered visual experience, imaginary or constructed visual experiences, auditory experience, and kinesthetic memories.[7,10-12] These clinical techniques offer such profound rapport and helpful clues to the student of nonverbal communication that patients often comment that they believe some extrasensory perception must be at work! In fact, the extraordinary effectiveness of this technique relies on extra attention to very ordinary sensory processes.

Once deep rapport has been established, it is necessary to address the features commonly associated with psychogenic voice disorders. These were described in detail in Chapter 9. The features which are a focus of clinical attention include anxiety in its many manifestations, time relationship to an event of acute stress or prolonged stress, the relationship of the stress and anxiety to interpersonal relationships, overcommitment, failure to set appropriate personal limits, inhibition about expressing views, anger or experiencing conflict over speaking out, and feelings of helplessness and powerlessness surrounding the ability to change.

One effective method for exploring these features utilizes the Gestalt techniques of awareness, exaggeration of physical behavior or significant statements, and enactment. An exploration of the secondary gain of the behavior is essential so that the individual's needs will be more adaptively met. When this is not undertaken, the patient often will experience symptom substitution. This is especially true in the profound psychogenic dysphonia which constitutes conversion disorder. Although interpretations are sometimes necessary to solidify insights patients acquire, any time the therapist offers his or her own conceptualization or instructions, the intervention is less effective. The patient is gently but firmly returned to his or her own resources to independently develop alternative solutions.

Six-step reframing derives from NLP and is a useful component of treatment for many psychological difficulties. Deep trance is not usually necessary. The altered state of deeply internal focused awareness develops as a result of the procedure itself. In this process, the therapist simply serves as a consultant for the patient's conscious mind, and the patient does the work him- or herself. The therapist communicates directly only with the patient's consciousness and instructs it how to proceed. The patient then takes the responsibility of establishing and maintaining effective communication with the unconscious portions that need to be accessed in order to change. Reframing is a specific way of contacting the "part" of the individual that is causing a certain behavior to occur or that is preventing a certain other behavior from occurring.[10] Central to the notion of reframing is the distinction between the intention of the behavior and the behavior itself. Once the intention (the secondary gain) has been brought into consciousness, new and more adaptive strategies for satisfying the same need can be generated. The unconscious "part" which has been maintaining the maladaptive behavior, in this case psychogenic dysphonia, remains free to utilize that means of guaranteeing the patient's well-being unless and until equally effective new strategies are presented.

The six steps are as follows:

1. Identify the pattern to be changed;
2. Establish communication in consciousness with the part that is responsible for the pattern. (For example, "Will the part of me that maintains this pattern communicate with me in consciousness?") The patient seeks a sensory signal and then establishes the yes/no meaning of that signal;
3. Distinguish between the behavior and the intention of the part that is responsible for the behavior. (For example, "Would you be willing to let me know in consciousness what you are trying to do for me with this voice difficulty?") If the patient gets a yes sensory response, he or she then asks the part to communicate its intention;
4. Create alternative behaviors to satisfy the intention. At the unconscious level, the part of the patient that has maintained the voice problem communicates its attention to a "creative part" and then selects from the alternatives the creative part generates. Each time it selects an alternative (a minimum of three), it gives the yes signal;
5. Ask the part, "Are you willing to take responsibility for generating the three new alternatives in the appropriate external context?"
6. Ecological check. "Is there any other part of me that objects to the three new alternatives?" If there is a yes response, the pattern is recycled to step 2 and continued until there are no objections.[7,10,11]

Once the intention has been established and alternative suggestions generated, the functional components of psychogenic dysphonia are addressed. Commonly, the three alternative solutions address at least some of these problems. Cognitive and behavioral strategies are then employed to assist the patient in developing and practicing a more adaptive behavioral repertoire. These include uncovering negative cognitions and implementing specific techniques designed to create cognitive and behavioral change. For example, recording thoughts prior to, during, and after an event; questioning the nonproductive nature of certain types of worry; confronting catastrophic thinking (and the use of "musts" and "shoulds"); and training in positive self-talk.[22] Anxiety and stress management training also are employed. A psychoeducational model is chosen for this, and patients are taught about the physiologic symptoms and effects of anxiety and inadequate responses to chronic stress. These were described in Chapter 15.

The importance of physical relaxation is stressed. Generalized progressive muscular relaxation involving the whole body is employed in the first session, and techniques that "scan" for target areas of muscle tension, especially in the head and neck, are components of all hypnotic interventions. Initially, this self-observation is prescribed hourly, and visual and auditory cues such as stickers or wristwatch timers may be helpful in the initial phases. A variety of hypnotic induction techniques is employed; and ordinarily audiotapes of these sessions are made for the patient's personal use. One very effective NLP modification is the use of visual-kinesthetic dissociation. Patients are invited to "Float up out of your body to a safe and amusing perch somewhere in the room . . . . Now, look down at him (her) and notice how he (she) looks, sounds, the state of relaxation of the muscles, the aroma and tastes which surround him (her), if any . . . . From that different point of view, gather information and develop ideas about how to correct any tensions and fulfill any unexpressed needs . . . . and when you are ready . . . . when you have learned all you can for now . . . . just float back down and rejoin her (him) in your body . . . . and make any and all adjustments that are in your best interest."

If, in self-monitoring of thoughts and internal self-talk, the patient notices that there are specific negative thoughts or images which are causing anxiety, the therapist encourages questioning of both the validity and necessity of such thoughts and images and their replacement with positive alternatives. Patients are encouraged to ask such questions as: "What is the evidence that supports or refutes my thoughts?" "What alternative perspectives exist?" "What is the effect of thinking the way I do?" "What errors of thinking am I making?" (including such things as all or nothing thinking, concentrating on weaknesses, and forgetting strengths, expecting perfection, exaggerating) and "What action can I take?" Thoughts are seen as hypotheses that should be challenged or tested, and abandoned if unproven. Patients learn to develop a number of positive, refuting statements about their success and worthiness.[22,23]

Difficulties with family and interpersonal relationships are the most common life stresses in association with psychogenic voice disorder and often include anxiety surrounding the expression of personal opinions or views and overcommitment. For example, some patients assume the burden of responsibility in their families because they lack sufficient assertiveness skills to set limits. Family therapy frequently is helpful as an adjunct in treatment of these patients. Because intervention as part of the voice treatment team has a brief mandate, family members may be reticent to attend; and the therapist is usually forced to work independently with the patient. Therapists who have the capability of providing longer term treatment would be well advised to probe for dysfunctional family dynamics and to address them as a focus of treatment.

Role playing in areas where the patient is finding communication difficult and training in assertiveness skills are frequently necessary. Many of these patients equate assertiveness with aggressiveness. Sometimes merely reiterating the definition of assertiveness, that is, standing up for one's legitimate rights and feelings in ways that do not abridge the rights or feelings of others offers some relief. The classic dilemma is well known to practicing psychotherapists. Patients who have difficulty with assertive communication often have trouble with individuation and the belief that they have legitimate rights at all.

As the patient learns to set limits, it is often helpful to reexamine a log of internal, negative self-talk and to engage in the exercise of refuting each statement with its positive antithesis. Strategies to help patients make changes that alter their life situation so that overcommitment and overinvolvement are decreased restore a sense of control. Enhancement of the individual's sense of personal efficacy has been shown to play a role in diminishing both depressive and anxiety disorders.[27]

RESPONSE TO VOCAL INJURY

Vocal injury in the professional voice user perceived as voice loss is usually seen as a challenge or loss of a primary life goal. It is unanticipated, may have been unexplained, and lasts for an indeterminate length of time, therefore creating overwhelming stress and testing normal coping mechanisms. At the time of diagnosis, it is an acute crisis, but it may not be immediately resolved and thus becomes an ongoing stressor. In this text, perceived or actual voice loss in this patient population has been compared to the series of emotional reactions typical of other grief and crisis experiences.

One common reaction to the feelings of helplessness and peril is anger because the patient has lost control over his or her life choices and body. The anger may be directed outward toward physicians, voice teachers, directors, families, friends, or God; or it may be reflected inward and result in guilt or depression. Anger also may be a response to the associated medical procedures or the insensitive comments of friends and family. These patients often feel isolated and benefit from participation in group psychotherapeutic interventions, as previously described. The guilt experience is particularly problematic. Many patients describe feeling responsible for the vocal injury even when a full explanation of the pathophysiology has been given. Performers blame themselves for decisions they have made in the past and sometimes feel they are being punished for some unknown past infraction.

When the anger is directed inward, depression is common and is considered a natural response to legitimate feelings of sadness and grief. These episodes usually are brief and periodic, but the mental health professional on the voice care team is responsible for ongoing vigilance regarding symptom intensity or persistence.

Perceived or actual loss of the voice may result in the loss of status, prestige, and self-image because of the expectations of the performer and his or her occupational and social network. It also may lead the patient to believe that his or her body is defective or damaged, resulting in feelings of inadequacy. An associated major loss is loss of control: these patients may no longer feel confident or competent. They are unable to plan their immediate or long-range futures and may lose financial security, as well as predictability and a sense of fairness about life in general.

During this grief response, there is predictable and concurrent mourning of all of the secondary losses experienced as consequences of the vocal injury. The depth of tragedy may not be recognized externally because the loss is one of potential, and others often do not understand the intensity of the pain. Schneider's work highlights that losses not recognized by outsiders; the "quiet tragedies" are more complicated to integrate psychologically than obvious and observable losses.[28] When voice impairment is permanent, the pain may lessen as time passes, life adjustments take place, and coping skills improve. Yet, the loss may never be completely resolved. Acceptance and adaptation may be more realistic.

Medical procedures necessary to diagnose and treat the vocal injury also may contribute to the crisis. These are additional stressors when the procedure itself is physically or psychologically stressful. For example, anesthesiologists or other medical care providers may be insensitive to psychological responses, provide inadequate information, or inflict discomfort. Some patients may demonstrate claustrophobic reactions during imaging studies. Many patients lack knowledge about normal psychological responses to acute or prolonged crisis. The clinician must provide information which normalizes the common emotional experiences and the attendant secondary losses. This validates the patient's pain and emotional suffering, and "unacceptable" affect, such as anger. Using the theoretical premises described in Chapter 10, the unique meaning of the vocal injury to the individual is assessed. The developmental impact of the voice on the patient's self-concept is explored through introspection. Gestalt techniques of enactment are particularly helpful in developing awareness of the profound emotion interwoven with these personal truths and facilitating its catharsis. Each psychotherapist will operate within the framework he or she believes to be most efficacious for this phase of therapy.

The psychological clinician is responsible for monitoring and facilitating the tasks of mourning. The intrapsychic processes of grieving move through an initial awareness of loss to modes of coping designed to distract or to limit the awareness of what has been lost. Any time human psychological adaptation is required, a part of the self tends to resist the change and simultaneously wishes to adapt and move on, divesting behaviors that are no longer functional. This has been described as the basic reaction of the human organism to loss and change. The two sides represent a profound ambivalence about facing the reality of loss. As the patient is helped to learn adaptive behaviors, he or she begins to let go of the past and begin the process of reaccumulating the energy attached to those things that have been lost. The therapist provides information about the normalcy of responses during grief and uses a variety of psychotherapeutic interventions to encourage the expression of a full range of grieving affects, most especially those which seem unacceptable or appear to be "split-off." Patients who become profoundly mentally disorganized need to be treated with protocols appropriate to their diagnosis, including the use of medication when the risk-benefit equation requires it.

Attention to holistic caretaking, including nutrition, hydration, rest, social contact, sexuality, spirituality, and the use of psychoactive substances should be specifically addressed. Pathologic grieving is less likely to occur when the initial reactive behaviors to loss are normalized and emotions fully expressed. The therapist may need to educate significant others in the patient's life who are encouraging denial as a means of protecting the patient from the pain of grief. Family members and significant others also may need instruction in the signs that the patient is no longer grieving adaptively and has become immobilized in depression or pathologic grief. Such patients should be immediately referred for professional intervention.

The point at which attempts to deny the loss fail is known as the *awareness phase*, and it is clearly the most painful, lonely, helpless, and hopeless time people face in their lives. Awareness usually comes unexpectedly when a stimulus triggers a memory that reminds the patient of the loss. At these moments, the patient is defenseless against the reality of his or her loss, and there is a flooding of consciousness with feelings of deprivation and the implications of the loss in daily life. These may be experienced physically and are commonly known as the "pangs" of grief. They may be accompanied by tightness in the throat, difficulty sleeping, intense and excruciating pain, deep sighing, weeping, or sobbing. The body literally aches for that which is lost. The intensity of feelings is greatest during this phase of the grieving process, and many patients report that they never believed they could endure so much.

Although losing something important terminates a significant portion of the patient's life, it does not necessarily finish what is important for him or her. What patients fear most is the incompleteness of their lives. Tension results from not being able to finish or resolve something critically important to them. This unfinished business, the unreached goals and the fantasies of the future, allows people to go on because they still desire to find ways in which they can manifest their professional identities. Slowly and often painfully, patients emerge from the exhausting phase of awareness, and other thoughts and activities begin to occupy more and more of their time.

Gradually, the pain lessens, and the pangs of awareness begin to ebb. This is often a time spent quietly and alone. Many patients listen to music which resonates their feelings or read reflective poetry or comforting books. The beauty of nature can also be restful and restorative. The support of trusted friends who are able to sit comfortably in silence or to touch is inestimable.

Healing is a painfully slow process, and it takes enormous energy to overcome the inertia that has accumulated during the acute phases of grief. Gaining perspective, being able to understand the loss and find its meaning in life, can come only from remaining open to the pain of grief and allowing the perspective to emerge. Anne Morrow Lindbergh wrote, "Patience, patience, patience is what the sea teaches. Patience and faith. One must lie empty, open, choiceless as a beach—waiting for a gift from the sea."[29(p17)]

Patients grow impatient with their grief and may also become fearful of it. They begin to answer the urge to get back to life as usual. The individual may need time alone to discover the healing that comes from being free of some of the demands of everyday life. With the acceptance of a new perspective comes a sense of peace. Some aspect of the loss no longer causes pain, and there may also be a sense of relief. The process of grieving is enormously stressful and may leave its mark physically, as well. There is a need for quiet rest and physical recuperation. In some patients, the loss is stored in some aspect of body memory and may be inadvertently triggered by touch, especially the therapeutic touch of massage or chiropractic adjustment. The emotional intensity begins to soften, as well.

In therapy, the clinician assists the grieving patient to acknowledge both the extent and the limits of his or her responsibility for the loss itself and for behaviors in reaction to the loss. However, it is important for clinicians to be aware that there is relatively little that they can do to facilitate the process of gaining perspective. Listening, encouraging self-trust, encouraging mourners to take time and space for self-reflection, and counseling the limitation of additional pressures may be most beneficial. The Gestalt grief trilogy is an invaluable component of intervention in the grief cycle. An active phase of saying goodbye is important. In this technique, enactment is utilized. In one formulation, the lost object, in this case the voice, is cradled in a chair; and the patient alternately expresses his or her resentments, appreciations, and regrets. Another variation involves the use of three chairs set at angles to one another; the patient sits in each of the chairs and speaks, "I am your resentments." These are then described; and in another, "I am your appreciation"; and in a third, "I am your regrets." The attendant emotional catharsis is supported and allowed to continue until the patient demonstrates that is complete. At that point, the therapist asks, "Are you ready to say goodbye?" If the answer is yes, the patient is encouraged to begin a soliloquy or eulogy in which he or she says goodbye to that which has been lost. If the answer is no, the patient is instructed to "go inside and receive counsel about what you may still need to do in order to feel ready to say goodbye." The therapy then proceeds to address the residual needs.

The final task of mourning, making meaningful the meaningless, begins when the patient is again able to feel centered within, feel balanced and able to focus on the present, and flow with whatever happens as it happens. Schneider calls this "a time of challenging all beliefs and developing an enduring sense of self-trust based on the capacity to deal with any life crisis without violating a personal sense of integrity. It is the time of exploring the possible instead of the improbable."[26(p226)] It is a time of new freedom and independence. The result of such a process of reformulation can be a level of openness that affects all life experiences.

One task of the psychotherapist caring for professional voice users who have experienced significant voice loss is to assist them in the process of grieving, as they disengage their sense of self *as* the voice and redefine themselves. It represents the general challenge of defining ourselves not for what we do, but for who we are. Who we are, however, is life's existential challenge. Psychological professionals who choose to care for this patient population accompany patients on the journey, remaining sensitive, respectful, and profoundly aware that the patient is engaged in defining the meaning of his or her life.

VOICE SURGERY

Patients who require voice surgery belong in the category of the voice injury. Some of these patients do not see themselves as professional voice users because they are not performers. However, our experience with performers has encouraged the view that all patients with voice injury are at psychological risk. Voice injury impairs the most familiar means by which human beings communicate, and an altered voice affects the way an individual is perceived by others. Chapter 11 reviewed in detail the role of the psychological professional and the preoperative assessment and some of the postoperative management of the patient who is scheduled to undergo voice surgery. Patients who demonstrate phobic responses to anesthesia or surgery often can be effectively treated by hypnotic approaches for short-term management of phobia.

The postoperative care of these patients involves the management of anxiety about the surgical outcome and occasionally dissatisfaction. This may occur even when the surgery has been "technically perfect" and vocal improvement is demonstrated on objective voice measures. It is particularly problematic in patients who have a less than perfect healing response. They need permission to express their disappointment and anger and to begin the process of adjusting to the new voice and grieving the loss of the old voice. The medical psychologist also may be involved in addressing treatment compliance involving not only cessation of behaviors that are injurious, but willingness to follow prescribed regimens for medication, speaking voice and singing voice exercises, and voice rest. The research of Rogers and Reich[30] has provided a schematic understanding of compliance and its competing demands on the patient. A trade-off exists between short-term difficulties of compliance (but future health) and the benefits of noncompliance, but poor prognosis. Other psychological issues such as borderline personality disorder, impaired family dynamics, marginal hope for cure, and resentment of the physician undergird noncompliant behavior.[30] This population responds especially well to treatment using a group psychotherapy model.

VOCAL TRACT CARCINOMA

Some patients will develop cancer. This consists of carcinoma of the vocal tract, adjacent aerodigestive structures, or distant sites. These individuals are forced to make major psychological and social adjustments. These include those related to a diagnosis of cancer; and when the cancer affects the vocal tract, of sudden impairment and disability: loss of voice. Psychological professionals participate in the care of these patients as adjunctive members of the treatment team. They may be found as part of the voice care team, in community practice, or as inpatient and outpatient care providers in hospitals offering cancer treatment.

Not every physical illness can be cured. Dr. Bernie Siegel is among the most well respected proponents of the view that all humans can make use of all illness to help redirect their lives.[31] Illness or suffering can lead to both intra- and interpersonal psychological growth. We are all dying, but some of us are aware of our death trajectory. Accepting mortality as a motivator and looking into the shadows of life summons new sources of self-esteem and self-love. The goal is not only length of days, but the quality of life. Karl Menninger in *The Vital Balance* writes, "It is our duty as physicians to estimate probabilities and to discipline expectations; but leading away from probabilities there are paths of possibility, towards which it is also our duty to hold aloft the light, and the name of that light is hope,"[32(p117)] or, to put it more simply, to cure sometimes, to control often, to comfort and console always.

Many professionals believe that psychological factors play a role in cancer onset and progression, and the popular media has promoted the writing and seminars of such experts as Bernie Siegel, Carl and Stephanie Simonton, and Gerald Jampolsky. Outcome studies of the scientific evidence supporting a relationship between physiological factors and cancer do not universally support those conclusions. This may be due to the complexities involved in studying cancer because of the multiple factors contributing to onset and progression, and also to methodological flaws. Levenson and Bemis reviewed the literature on cancer onset and progression.[33] In tracking epidemiologic conclusions, they reviewed studies on cancer onset and progression as affected by psychological variables, and psychological factors impacting the immune system. The variables examined included affective states, coping/defensive styles and personality traits, interpersonal variables, and stressful life events. The research concluded that, "a number of studies have lent some support to the relationship between a variety of psychological factors and the onset, exacerbation, or outcome of neoplastic disease," but no absolute associations or causal relationships had been proven.[33(p92)] More recent, less flawed studies have suggested that cancer progression, rather than onset, may be influenced by psychosocial factors. Better, systematically designed research is sorely needed.

One major concern involves the potential delay in state-of-the-art diagnosis and treatment protocols which have favorable statistical outcomes when patients select only alternative approaches. Many of the leaders currently espousing attitudinal healing are also physicians. None of them suggests delaying or refusing traditional treatment; rather, they offer information about the benefits of combining traditional and adjunctive approaches to care. Beliefs about cancer onset and progression may not be supported empirically, but they nonetheless can contribute to the patient's sense of well-being and control.

Early procedures for attitude assessment in patients with cancer caused some professionals to conclude that patients were being held responsible for their diseases because of "poor attitudes" or personality characteristics, and these have been modified. All of these directions of inquiry assist patients in understanding the potential secondary gain of their characteristic coping styles (usually lack of assertiveness, lack of self-care, and lack of personal boundaries) in their lives. Once these components have been identified, therapy can focus on ways to meet those needs more adaptively; and psychic energy is released for more active participation in the treatment process.

The reader is referred to the excellent text *Psychosocial Factors Affecting Medical Conditions* for specific, detailed reports and criticisms of the available research.[33] One study will be mentioned by way of example. Spiegel[34,35] and colleagues randomly assigned breast cancer patients with metastases to 1 year of psychosocial treatment consisting of weekly supportive group therapy and training in self-hypnosis for pain control. The control group received routine oncologic care. At 1 year, the psychotherapy treatment group had less mood disturbance and fewer phobic responses, and half as much pain. At 10-year follow-up, the mean survival time was 34.8 months for the group randomized to psychotherapy as opposed to 18.9 months for the control group. The authors stated that they had expected to, and did, find a beneficial effect of treatment on mood, but had not expected that psychosocial treatment would affect survival.[34,35]

Simonton[36] et al have written that, because cancer is such a dreaded disease, the moment people learn of a cancer diagnosis, it becomes the patient's defining characteristic regardless of the numerous roles he or she ordinarily plays. Therefore, the person's full human identity is lost to his or her cancer identity, and all treatment is aimed at the patient as a body, not as a person. The psychotherapist will be one of the members of the team who responds to the patient's other roles: parent, spouse, lover, sibling, child, boss, friend, as well as to the numerous personal characteristics such as intelligence, humor, charm, and sensitivity. An imperative of psychological management in a cancer diagnosis is the central premise that illness is not purely a physical problem, but rather a problem of the whole person: body, mind, emotions, and spirituality. So, responsible care (which may or may not offer cure) requires that we consider not only what is happening to the individual on a physical level but, just as importantly, what is occurring in the rest of the patient's life.

Dilts[13] describes beliefs and belief systems as one of the frameworks for behavior. When a patient truly believes something, he or she will behave congruently with that belief, positive or negative. The first type of belief is called *outcome expectancy*. In relationship to health, it means that the patient believes it is possible for someone to recover from a disease. Conversely, when patients do not believe that a goal is possible, they respond with hopelessness and do not take the appropriate actions for recovery. The placebo effect is one example of *response expectancy*, that is, what one expects to happen, either positively or negatively, as a result of actions taken in a particular situation. Beliefs usually are not based on a logical framework of ideas and are notoriously unresponsive to logic. Patients will hold many types of beliefs. Among them are beliefs about cause, beliefs about the meaning of events, and beliefs about identity, including boundaries and personal limits.[13] The techniques described by Robert Dilts, as well as his colleagues Halbom and Smith, are particularly effective in helping patients examine both limiting and enhancing beliefs. In addition, their work refines some of the traditional visualization techniques in ways that increase their effectiveness. Practitioners of Ericksonian hypnosis and NLP will recognize the addition of association and submodality modification to customary techniques. Their research revealed that generating a well-formed outcome, visualizing a fully associated experience of that outcome, and adding the submodalities of expectation improved the statistical success of visualization. The work of Siegel and Simonton has provided lay access to techniques of introspection (What is the illness helping me to learn about myself and my needs?), the addition of expressive modalities such as art and music, and the value of hypnosis for relaxation and enhancement of well being throughout cancer treatment.

Siegel[31] also writes eloquently about the role of the professional who chooses to work with cancer patients. He quotes an oncologist colleague who describes the many gifts which flow from the patient to caregivers who are comfortable receiving them. "From my perspective, it seems that the peace we see in some cancer patients involves being willing to give up life as we normally perceive it and view life only as a moment-by-moment occurrence of opportunities to give love. In the giving of love, there is also the receiving of love, and this cycle continues without bounds."[31(p151)] A medical student pursuing a fellowship with Siegel described his intrapersonal struggle with the notion of being available to patients with life-threatening illness to the very end of their treatment. "It is important to come to an acceptance of death, not only as an absolute reality, but as part of the natural order of things. When the physician achieves this acceptance, he or she no longer needs to avoid people who have problems he or she cannot solve. The physician is then able to remain in a partnership with the patient and to share the common bond of mortality that they have between them until the very end. As George Santayana has said, 'There is no cure for birth and death save to enjoy the interval'."[31(p233)]

Only through the acceptance of mortality and love can we enjoy the interval. These admonitions apply equally to providers of psychological care throughout the experience of cancer. Hemingway wrote, "The world breaks everyone, and afterward many are stronger at the broken places."[37] Both the challenges and the rewards of providing care to this population are enormous. Not everyone will choose to undertake this work, but those who do will find themselves examining the very core of themselves. We need not have all the answers, merely the willingness to seek them *with* the patient and the courage to stay present and in full contact until the end of our work together, whenever that may be. Elie Wiesel, whose extraordinary wisdom was forged as a result of his experiences in the Holocaust, writes, "When we die and go to heaven and we meet our Maker, our Maker is not going to say to us, Why didn't you become a Messiah? Why didn't you discover the cure for such and such? The only thing we are going to be asked at that precious moment is, Why didn't you become fully you?"[38(p241)]

STRESS MANAGEMENT/PERFORMANCE ANXIETY

Chapter 15 discussed in detail concepts of stress theory and the physiologic effects of extraordinary and/or chronic stress on the human body. The negative and positive benefits of coping styles on psychological and somatic distress also have been described in several chapters. The psychological professional frequently will receive as referrals from physicians, speech-language pathologists, voice teachers, music teachers, and acting coaches patients whose level of stress and/or inadequate stress response style are producing poor outcomes.

One of the first tasks, after engaging these individuals in treatment and negotiating a mutual contract, is the assessment of the individual's life experience and previous coping styles. Every clinician will have a favored method for accomplishing this. In an initial session, we recommend a psychoeducational approach, describing stress theory and its biophysical effects. Patients usually volunteer significant amounts of information, both verbally and nonverbally, during such a discussion. Charts and diagrams are used to reinforce understanding, and ordinarily copies of these are provided for patients' personal review. As the session concludes, self-assessment tasks are assigned to be prepared before the next session. A number of commercially available tools exist for this purpose and are occasionally used. Patients in our clinical practice often are given the materials included in Appendix I, including the drawing tasks.

At the second session, the patient and psychotherapist review these tools in detail. An informal interview allows patients to amplify significant areas, and the clinician can support the expression of emotion associated with them. Based on the individual responses provided, the psychotherapist designs or reviews a number of categories of stress skills. Four basic approaches, described in the following way, are utilized:

1. Reorganize yourself to take better control of the way you spend time and energy.
2. Manage your environment by controlling who and what surrounds you.
3. Change you attitude towards your stressors.
4. Build-up your physical and emotional strength and endurance.

Every human being develops favorite ways of coping; and because they have worked in the past, people continue trying to cope with methods that no longer work for a multiplicity of reasons. The psychotherapist challenges patients to enhance their flexibility and to consider using, in a time-limited way, some unfamiliar or underdeveloped strategies. They can, of course, revert to their customary approaches; and the principle of "prescribing the symptom" implies that therapists would do well to suggest that this is expected to happen, so that patients do not devalue themselves further for perceived failure.

Under the strategy of *organizing oneself,* the patient and clinician consider the art of choosing between alternatives and determining which is more worthwhile. This helps determine the ways in which time is spent based on the patient's personal values. Many patients either have not learned the skill of planning or have become so overwhelmed that they no longer do so effectively. Once patients learn a strategy for defining what they wish to accomplish, designing a program for getting there is much simpler. Once a goal is established and behaviors to achieve it are recorded, one must commit and invest him- or herself in the outcome. This is risky, but life without commitment is unrewarding.

Time management is critical to the concept of stress management, and many patients allow time to slip away without accomplishing what they most desire. Time management skills help to reduce waste time and make use of even 5- or 10-minute periods throughout the day to accomplish tasks which have been "chunked down." Patients are asked to take an 8½ × 11 piece of paper and divide it into 7 days of the week on the vertical axis and 24 hours in each day on the horizontal axis. They then write in everything that they are currently doing in one typical week and, using crayons, transparent markers, or colored pencils in three different colors, select one shade for the "must do," another shade for the "should do," and a third shade for the "would like to do" categories. The patient and psychologist consider together whether the solid lines defining the time spent could be realistically turned into interrupted lines, allowing more time flexibility. A discussion of pacing, controlling the internal tempo, is conducted. The skill of pacing allows steady, even progress and diminishes the wear and tear of stress. This will include a repertoire of speeds for a variety of occasions and demands.

The second approach, *changing scene,* means changing the way the patient relates to people around him or her. Often, overstressed people lack supporting relationships, although they may have contact with or experience demands from an excessive number of individuals. Psychological work focuses on elements of contact, including reaching out to those who can help to increase the patient's energy via self-disclosure, feedback, and appropriate choices of the proper individual for each unique need. Relationships are more mutual when the people in them are skilled in the art of empathy. Sometimes, patients need assistance in learning to tune in to the feelings of others and respond to them. The stress relief of long-term, lasting relationships in which individuals can be honestly themselves and freely exchange feelings of all types is enhanced by developing the skill of empathy.

One recurring problem for patients with poor stress management techniques is lack of assertiveness. Assertive communication skills, enabling the individual to say no when he or she wants to say no, are taught and practiced through role playing. Occasionally, self-esteem demands fighting for what one believes in. When this is identified as a concern, patients learn to choose their fights carefully and to fight fair. Flight can also be positive, and people need to know when and how to retreat and find a safe haven. Both actual physical escape and the ability to use relaxation and hypnotic strategies are skills that are components of stress management therapy.

A third approach, *changing one's point of view,* addresses the cognitive distortions which very often characterize poor stress management strategies. Homework assignments in the identification of dysfunctional thoughts and then refuting with the skills of positive self-talk are critical. Reframing (relabeling with a more positive term for each stressor) requires looking for the promise in every problem and gaining wider perspective. Sometimes patients need to learn when to let go and let be. For perfectionistic, ambitious, self-made individuals, this set of attitudes or behaviors becomes equated with giving up. Some life forces will be bigger than any individual. Sometimes the surrender of accepting the present and acknowledging personal limitations is of vital importance.

Human beings vary in their acceptance of a spiritual dimension, but life includes the mysterious and the unknowable; and this dimension, when patients can include it in their lives, helps them to deal with the stress that results from confronting existential questions. No helping professional should engage in religious proselytizing, but gentle, respectful questions about patients' spiritual or philosophical beliefs can invite them to consider ritual and old or new traditions as sources of support in their lives.

Humor! It is no accident that our lexicon abounds with the cliches surrounding humor. Laughter frequently *is* the best medicine for a world of reality that is often inconsistent. It is probably impossible to install a sense of humor where none has ever existed, but merely observing the ironies of life can permit most people to use the perspective of the ridiculous. Most therapists skilled in the use of visualization have had the opportunity to suggest a tension-producing scene and then add an auditory dimension of circus music. This often has an effect comparable to releasing the end of an overfilled balloon and watching it sail erratically around the room, making obnoxious noises. One simply cannot feel the same afterward.

Humans talk to themselves internally virtually all of the time, and it is just as easy to be speaking messages of love, validation, and support as it is to produce the self-destructive and judgmental beliefs of limiting introjects. This is one of the most basic elements of the cognitive therapy approach. Finally, in conjunction with the patient's physicians, the psychological professional encourages physical strength and stamina by more healthful behaviors. This usually includes exercise within any medically imposed limits, nutrition, and hydration including the completion and mutual review of food diaries, sufficient sleep, and relaxation skills.

Regular use of strategies for deep relaxation and visualization have well-established medical and psychological benefits. In clinical practice, at least one lengthy hypnotic induction, deepened with instructions for progressive muscle relaxation, is conducted. This is followed by the installation of an image of the patient's personally selected "safe haven" and a visual, auditory, kinesthetic, and olfactory/gustatory experience of safety and well-being. The trance experience is concluded with posthypnotic suggestions for brief self-induction. The entire process is recorded on audiotape and provided to the patient. Self-hypnotic induction and emergence are practiced, and appropriate uses of brief moments of deep relaxation and positive visualization at frequent intervals throughout the day are described. Patients often choose to use this as part of a sleep hygiene approach to insomnia.

Stress is value neutral. Selye coined the term eu-stress and contrasted it with distress to reinforce his theory that it is what each individual *does* with personal stressors which makes the difference in physiologic response and long-term consequences.[39] To be effective, stress management strategies, must be accepted. Acceptance requires that these strategies be individually designed and maintain respect for the positive role of stress in maintaining the "edge" in highly skilled performers of all fields. Chapter 15 describes current psychological thinking in the area of performance anxiety. Regardless of the psychotherapist's theoretical orientation, all clinicians who work in the area of arts medicine concur that performance anxiety is a widespread and serious problem among performers in all fields.

Clinical approaches to the treatment of performance anxiety parallel theoretical understanding about the cognitive schemas that establish negative self-evaluation initially and the cognitive, affective and behavioral responses that serve to maintain it. In addition, unconscious psychological needs which are met by the avoidance of performance often will continue to interfere with the gains patients make using brief, directed, cognitive and behavioral treatment approaches. For this reason, it is critical to use an integrated approach during treatment planning and care. In the authors' practice, this concept is discussed with patients as soon as rapport allows it to be empathically introduced. Many of the areas to consider are painful. Performance anxiety has a positive intention in the life of the affected performer. Its method of offering that kind of protection, however, causes enormous suffering. All clinicians will utilize their own theoretical training as they assist patients to explore for these areas of conflict. Some will offer treatment using psychodynamic interpretation; others may select Gestalt enactment techniques. The cognitive and/or rational-emotive strategies of examining catastrophic thinking may be beneficial, as well. All of these are means to discovering beliefs, the highly valued negative and positive criteria which undergird the life of each individual.

The six-step reframing procedure described in the section on psychogenic dysphonia is frequently useful in examining the positive intention of performance anxiety. This can also be elucidated with a series of questions. For example, "What does your performance anxiety buy for you?" If the patient gives up his or her "addiction" to the problem, what might be expected, and where might that lead? Patients will have to answer the question, "Am I ready to go on?" Sometimes these answers surface a degree of awareness that problems with performing ensure a comfortable anonymity instead of a challenging career. They may highlight intrapersonal conflicts regarding the performer's self-concept and sense of entitlement to satisfaction and fulfillment. Conflict regarding competition may also be uncovered. Ristad's text, *A Soprano on Her Head*, includes a delightful visualization which can be successfully accomplished with or without preliminary hypnosis.[14]

Barry Green has applied the "inner game" techniques of W. Timothy Gallwey to music.[40] In the authors' practice, instruction and experiments with the techniques described in his text have been extremely successful. Green addresses the theoretical notion of self-interference in a simple and direct fashion. He invites the reader to, "Take a moment to think about the things that make you nervous, and imagine yourself going on stage to perform feeling all those last-minute anxieties. Make a mental list of all the things that worry you." Participants in his research listed these commonalities: doubt of their own ability, fears they would lose control, feelings that they hadn't practiced enough, concern they wouldn't see or hear properly, worry about their accompanist, thoughts that their equipment might malfunction, worry about losing their place in the music, doubt that the audience would like their playing, fear they would forget what they had memorized, or fear that, even if everything went well, their parents would still be disappointed they hadn't gone into another career.

These doubts and fears crop up in everyone who performs, regardless of the venue. The physical and mental effects of doubt and anxiety during performance were previously elucidated. They result from the outpouring of epinephrine and other catacholamines as a result of the mobilization of the body's response to threat. These include the "fight or flight" and the "freeze or faint" responses. The inner game philosophy applies the labels "self 1" and "self 2" to the competing internal dialogue which plays such a critical role in the mind-body connection. Gallwey refers to the voice doing the talking as "self 1" and person spoken to as "self 2." He calls "self 1" our interference, containing concepts about how things should be and all judgments and associations. "Self 2" consists of the vast reservoir of potential within each person and contains all natural talents and abilities; it serves as a resource, and without interference performs with gracefulness and ease.[40]

Children learn to walk and talk naturally, and they are avid learners. As humans mature, they begin to accumulate ideas and attitudes and incorporate the voices of authoritative others, also known as introjects. This is how belief is structured. These internal beliefs serve a positive function when they provide security about what we know and can take for granted. However, the loss of this "magical child" limits the open and absorbing attitudes of childhood. As we age, the gap between the critical and creative selves becomes wider and wider, and most adults lose their spontaneous ability to tap their inner resources and to play. Clinicians may find it efficacious to assist patients in forming visual images of their "judges" and confronting them.

In order to design personalized, effective therapeutic strategies, it is important for psychotherapists to understand how the patient uniquely structures his or her belief and how validating information is accessed and processed. The NLP techniques described in the section on rapport building are extremely useful in this task. The patient is asked to remember a time in the recent past when performance anxiety manifested itself. By merely observing the patient's physiology as that information is recalled, the astute hypnotherapist will notice concrete changes in the patient's rate and depth of respiration, muscle tone, skin color, eye focus and pupil dilatation, eye accessing cues, subtle gestures, and subvocalization. Effectiveness is greatly enhanced by "speaking the patient's language" in the use of predicates and by obtaining a full description of the patient's sensory experience in those situations.

We invite patients to "visualize their judges in a circle around us and to give them shape and form." For some people, the judges are abstract representations of malevolence; for others they are recognizable personalities, often authority figures from the patient's past. The patient is asked to visualize both of us standing in the center of the circle and to have an associated sensory experience by looking at each judge with a sense of detachment and curiosity and inviting each one to explain what we need to understand. The patient takes the initiative, instructing them to stop the tyranny. This enhances the patient's sense of control and improves limit setting. We can also collaborate with them and ask them to tell us or show us the positive intention of their commentary. This opportunity can be used to create incongruity and introduce humor or restructure the hierarchy. Ristad[14] described two patients, one of whom turned her judges into ice and then visualized a tiny warm glow in the center of her own body which melted the judges and caused them to trickle down a rocky slope and into a rushing stream which flowed all the way to the ocean. Another patient dressed her judges in judicial robes and then watched them grow Pinocchio-like noses as a brisk wind tore their robes to shreds, leaving them naked. This humorous representation of an alteration in the power structure robbed the judges of their power to inhibit her.

Some performers are also profoundly inhibited by their long-distance view of success. This is an unfortunate consequence of the training tradition used with talented young vocal and instrumental musicians; but ascribing success only to a destination is perilous. When human beings devote all of their energies to reaching the goal, they often block all simultaneous sensory experience of the journey. Ambition and discipline are reinforced by significant figures during that process. Distractions, diversion, and a more rounded definition of positive self-concept are seen as interferences with attaining virtuoso status. Unfortunately, once this superhuman performer arrives at success, all of the psychological and behavioral habits of the journey remain, and enjoyment of the pinnacle continues to be impaired by preparation for the next stretch of development. Whenever human beings apply themselves to one task to the exclusion of their senses, they miss the essence of perception and the value of conscious awareness and a wide horizon. According to Green, "self 2" performs best in an "unthinking state," one in which "we are relaxed yet aware, and are letting our ability and musicality express itself, without trying to control and manipulate it."[40(p21)]

Once a therapist has discovered the sensory structure of performance anxiety through the patient's description of the sensory experience and listened to the concomitant internal dialogue, strategies can be suggested. These are best used within a visualization which installs the antithetical response, neutralizing the prior experience. Almost every individual will *do* something internally that results in the discomfort. The physical responses are simply the consequences of how the patient's mind has created the sense of threat. The psychotherapist can directly change the elements of internal experience by noticing presuppositions and using verbal intervention to reframe the experience utilizing deeply held beliefs which counteract them. For example, a common belief among performers afflicted with disabling performance anxiety is that the audience knows more about all of the components of excellent performance than they do. The clinician might suggest, "OK, let me ask you something important. Do you believe that the knowledgeable people who come to hear you play (sing, act) would be so foolish as to pick a performance they believe to be inferior?" This leaves the patient with a double-bind or paradox. This is the premise underlying confusion induction, and the patient usually will drop briefly into an altered state during which integration of the new insight takes place.

The psychotherapist may choose to experiment with any of the sensory modalities or submodalities of the patient's experience, as well. For example, many people who are impaired by extreme performance anxiety experience it as a response to being watched, and this often takes the form of how they see the eyes or faces of audience members.[15] The therapist might suggest, "As you're standing up there on stage, look past the 'scrutinizing' eyes and see the 'music-loving' eyes of the people in your audience . . . Start with just one person, and when you can see those sensitive eyes, let your eyes move on to another face . . . and then another face. Continue to make eye contact with all the people . . . at your own rate and pace . . . and as your emotional experience changes, come back here, be with me, and tell me about the changes you have experienced." Therapists who are familiar with hypnotic techniques will note that this communication includes instructing the patient to have an associated experience and embeds the "yes set" that a positive change will occur within the patient's internal experience.

Patients who cannot generate a positive personal experience are instructed to summon the image of someone who does the desired behavior expertly. This person's skills are then studied in minute detail by the patient as an observer. Finally the patient is invited to, "'Step inside' that expert performer (associated experience) . . . and to see, hear, feel, taste, and smell what he or she does in that situation." The affective and physiologic experience of success in that role is then available to the patient. This connection is often strengthened by some tactile anchor in a spot on the body easily and unobtrusively accessible to the patient. The patient is then invited to, "Come back here, be with me, and describe and discuss the experience."

In *The Inner Game of Music*, three skills are highlighted: awareness, will, and trust. These skills combine to form "relaxed concentration" which offers balance between performance achievement, experience, and learning. *Awareness* is the fundamental skill. "When we are simply aware, without judgment, of the degree to which the outcome of our acts matches our intention, natural learning takes place."[40(p28)] When people employ judgment and try to figure out what went wrong, overcompensating for any error and tightening the muscles, more errors are produced. Gallwey defines *will*, the second inner game skill as, "Both the direction and intensity of intention."[40(p29)] Will sets the goal, moves directly toward it and then resets its sights to come closer to accomplishing the goal the next time. Will uses feedback from awareness to improve its aim. *Trust* is cited as the third of the inner game skills. Trust is necessary to allow awareness without immediately bombarding oneself with criticism and judgment. It also takes trust to use a trial-and-error approach and to tap into inner resources.[40] The essence of the inner game of music is developing these three skills and balancing them.

Psychotherapeutic management of disabling performance anxiety allows professionals to improve their artistry and regain their enjoyment of their craft. Early intervention during the education of performers and their teachers offers the possibility of avoiding this painful and disabling problem. Knowledge that help is available should prevent affected singers, actors, and public speakers from suffering in silence.

The psychological professional caring for performers with performance anxiety is in a key position to assist them to release the powerful restraining forces that inhibit their careers. We stand in awe of these gifted individuals, and it is indeed a privilege to allow their talent to flow freely once more.

Those of us who care for that uniquely human capability—the voice—quickly come to understand the essential role of psychological awareness in our treatment failures and successes. Contemporary medical care has come full circle with the teachings of the earliest physicians who were cautioned by Socrates that, "it is not proper to cure the eyes without the head, nor the head without the body, so neither is it proper to cure the body without the soul." The relationship between the mind and the body has intrigued physicians throughout the history of medicine, and assessing and supporting that relationship are the special province of the arts medicine psychologist providing care to performers with physical impairments.

REFERENCES

1. Nicholas D, Gobble D, Crose R, Frank B. A systems view of health, wellness, and implications for mental health counselling. *Journal of Mental Health Counseling*, 1992;14:8–17.
2. Morales A, Sheafor B. *Social work: a profession of many faces*. Allyn and Bacon Inc; Boston, Mass: 1977:1.
3. Sataloff RT. Proposal for establishing a degree of doctor of philosophy in arts medicine. *J Voice*. 1992;6(1):17–21.
4. Bady SL. The voice as a curative factor in psychotherapy. *Psychoanal Rev*. 1985; 72:479–490.
5. Crasilneck HB, Hall J. *Clinical Hypnosis: Principles and Applications*, 2nd ed. Orlando, Fla: Grune & Stratton; 1985;60–61.
6. Watkins J. *Hypnotherapeutic Techniques*. New York, NY: Irvington; 1987;114.
7. Lankton S. *Practical Magic: A Translation of Neuro-Linguistic Programming into Clinical Psycho-Therapy*. Cupertino, Calif: Meta; 1980:174.
8. King M, Novick L, Citrenbaum C. *Irresistible Communication*. Philadelphia, Pa: WB Saunders; 1983:21-22, 115–127.
9. Klein R. *A Certification Program in Ericksonian Techniques for Mental Health Professionals*. Silver Spring, Md: American Hypnosis Training Academy; 1988.
10. Bandler R, Grinder J. *Frogs into Princes: Neuro-Linguistic Programming*. Moab, Utah: Real People Press; 1979:5–78.
11. Bandler R. *Using Your Brain for a Change*. Moab, Utah: Real People Press, 1985:1–34.
12. Andreas C, Andreas S. *Heart of the Mind: Engaging Your Inner Power to Change*. Moab, Utah: Real People Press; 1989:1–84.
13. Diltz R. *Beliefs: Pathways to Health and Well Being*. Portland, OR: Metamorphous Press; 1990:12–45.
14. Ristad E. *A Soprano on her Head: Rightside Up Reflections on Life and Other Performances*. Moab, Utah: Real People Press; 1982:151–155.
15. Andreas C, Andreas S. *Heart of the Mind: Engaging Your Inner Power to Change*. Moab, Utah: Real People Press; 1989:1–7.
16. Tedeschi R, Calhoun L. Using the support group to respond to the isolation of bereavement. *J Ment Health Counsel*. 1993;15:47–54.
17. Carpenter B. *Psychological aspects of vocal fold surgery*. In Gould WJ, Sataloff RT, Spiegel JR, Voice Surgery. St. Louis, Mo: CV Mosby; 1993:342.

18. Walsh F, McGoldrick M. *Living Beyond Loss: Death in the Family.* New York, NY: WW Norton and Co; 1991:xviii.
19. Shakespeare W. MacBeth, Act V, Scene 3. In Wright WA ed. *The Complete Works of Shakespeare.* Garden City, NJ: Garden City Books; 1936:1052.
20. Malan DH. *Individual Psychotherapy and the Science of Psychodynamics.* London: Butterworths Press; 1979:74–94.
21. Rogers M, Reich P. Psychosomatic medicine and consultation liaison psychiatry. In Nicholi A ed. *The New Harvard Guide to Psychiatry.* Cambridge, Mass: Harvard University Press; 1988:387–417.
22. Butcher P, Elias A, Raven R. *Psychogenic Voice Disorders and Cognitive Behavior Therapy.* San Diego, Calif: Singular Publishing Group Inc, 1993:41, 58–150.
23. Beck A, Rush A, Snow B, Emery G. *Cognitive Therapy of Depression.* New York, NY: Guilford Press; 1979:87–103.
24. Beck A, Emery G. *Anxiety Disorders and Phobias.* New York, NY: Basic Books; 1985:19-53, 190–209.
25. Weisman A. *Coping with Cancer.* New York, NY: McGraw-Hill Press; 1979:409.
26. Amatea ES, Fong-Beyette ML. Through a different lens: examining professional women's inter-role coping by focus and mode. *Sex Roles.* 1987;17: 237–252.
27. Bandura A. Perceived self-efficacy and the exercise of personal agency. *The Psychologist.* 1989;2:411–424.
28. Schneider J. *Stress Loss and Grief.* Baltimore, Md: University Park Press; 1984:26.
29. Lindbergh AM. *Gift from the Sea.* New York, NY: Vantage Books; 1975:17.
30. Rogers M, Reich P. Psychosomatic medicine and consultational liaison psychiatry. In: Nicholi A ed. *The New Harvard Guide to Psychiatry.* Cambridge, Mass: Harvard University Press; 1988:411.
31. Siegel B. Peace, *Love and Healing: Body Mind Communication and the Path to Self-Healing.* New York, NY: Harper and Rowe; 1989:9–281.
32. Menniger K. *The Vital Balance: The Life Process in Mental Health and Illness.* Gloucester, Mass: Peter Smith Publisher; 1983:117.
33. Levenson J, Bemis C. *Cancer onset and progression. In: Stoudemire A. Psychological Factors Affecting Physical Condition.* Washington, DC: American Psychiatric Press Inc; 1995:81–93.
34. Spiegel D, Bloom JR, Yalem ID. Group support for patients with metastatic cancer: a randomized prospective outcome study. *Arch Gen Psy.* 1981;38: 527–533.
35. Spiegel D, Bloom JR, Kramer HC, et al. Effects of psychosocial treatment on survival of patients with metastatic breast cancer. *Lancet.* 1989;2:888–891.
36. Simonton OC, Stipes—, Mathews-Simonton S, Creighton JL. *Getting Well Again.* New York, NY: Bantam Books; 1980:10–20.
37. Hemingway E. *A Farewell to Arms.*
38. Wiesel E. *Souls on Fire.* New York, NY: Summit Books; 1972; As cited in: Siegel B. Peace, Love and Healing: Body Mind Communication and the Path to Self-Healing. New York, NY: Harper and Rowe; 1989:9–281.

39. Selye H. On the real benefits of eustress. *Psych Today.* 19—;12(10):60–64.
40. Green B. *The Inner Game of Music.* New York, NY: Doubleday; 1986:15–36.

CHAPTER

17

Perceived Voice Loss in Professional Voice Users: Principles and Case Studies With Guided Drawing Assignments

his chapter describes data derived from a pilot study designed to test the validity of a grief and loss framework in the evaluation and treatment of professional voice users who experience vocal impairment. Guided drawing assignments were utilized as one component of the assessment. The results of the study and related therapeutic experience have proven vital to the assessment of anecdotal observation and have guided the principles articulated in this textbook.

Perceived voice loss in this population was conceptualized as a crisis, and crisis was regarded as a "dangerous opportunity," that is, a situation in which the outcome holds, with equal probability, danger and opportunity. Individuals encounter situations which are defined as crisis according to their internalized, personal cognitive set. Each individual operates at a "functional baseline" in the cognitive, affective, and behavioral domains of his or her life. Crisis theory maintains that crisis response is, by definition, time-limited, rarely exceeding 6 weeks.[1] At the point of crisis resolution, there are three outcome possibilities. In the first, the patient returns to his or her precrisis functional baseline. In the second, the level of function deteriorates. In the third, the level of function improves; the individual grows from the experience. Crisis intervention research has provided evidence that these outcomes can be intervention-dependent, "premorbid" personality-dependent, history-dependent, and/or context-dependent. These outcomes are heavily dependent on the personal meaning of the crisis event to the patient and the presence of endogenous or exogenous stressors.

In Chapter 10, Response to Vocal Injury, the hypothesis that professional voice users who experience a serious threat to their vocal quality or stamina also experience a serious threat to self-definition and self-image was introduced. These patients experience grief which is similar to patients who mourn for other losses such as the death of a loved one. "Normal" grief, also known as "uncomplicated" grief, encompasses a broad range of feelings and behaviors which are common to individuals after loss. The initial work in this area was done by Lindemann in 1944 and reported in his classic paper "The Symptomatology and Management of Acute Grief."[2] Parks and Bowlby[3] expanded Lindemann's work with their research on the phases through which a mourner must pass before grief is finally resolved. In all of these models, there is overlap between the various phases, and they more often behave like a spiral.

The grief inventory administered to subjects in this study was modified from a list of manifestations of normal grief described under the four general categories of *affect, physical sensations, cognitions,* and *behaviors.* The responses endorsed by patients at each of their assessment sessions allow us to understand the degree to which their entire experience has been disordered by the perception (or reality) of the loss of a part of self: the voice.

In the domain of affect, sadness, anger, guilt and self-reproach, anxiety, loneliness, fatigue, helplessness, shock, yearning, numbness, emancipation, and relief are described. All of these are normal feelings, and they are pathological only when they exist for abnormally long periods of time or at excessive intensity. The physical sensations associated with acute grief reaction are often overlooked, but they are certainly significant for the mourner. Usually, patients need to be queried about their presence because they often fail to associate them with their reactions to loss. These sensations include hollowness in the stomach, tightness in the chest, tightness in the throat, oversensitivity to sensory stimulation, depersonalization, derealization, breathlessness, muscle weakness, lack of energy, and dry mouth. Cognitions are thoughts which appear and eventually disappear throughout the stages of grieving. Some of these thoughts, if they persist, increase the likelihood that a clinically evident mood disorder or anxiety disorder may result.

Among those patients have listed are disbelief, confusion, preoccupation, sense of presence, and hallucinations. Specific behaviors frequently associated with grief reactions are commonly reported. These may include sleep disturbance, appetite disturbance, confusion, social withdrawal, dreams of the lost object, avoiding reminders of the lost object, searching and calling out, sighing, restlessness, crying, and visiting places or carrying things which remind the griever of the lost object.[4]

Bowlby's[3] work suggests that all humans, regardless of their society or culture, grieve loss to one degree or another. Animals demonstrate changed behaviors after loss of their mates and offspring, as well. According to Bowlby's[3] work on attachment theory, in the course of evolution, instinctual equipment developed around the fact that the lost are sometimes retrievable. The behavioral responses that make up part of the grieving process are geared toward reestablishing relationship with the lost object.

The patients discussed in this chapter, and in most of the rest of our practice, did indeed manifest the responses characteristic of mourning after loss. In general, they moved through four phases: *shock and numbness,* followed by *searching and yearning,* deteriorating to *disorganization and despair* with difficulty functioning in the environment; and finally, in cases with sufficiently long follow-up, the phase of *reorganization.*[5] In bereavement research, these phases tend to occur at characteristic periods within the first year after loss in uncomplicated mourning. That is not to imply that grief is complete at the end of 12 months, but merely that, in many kinds of loss due to death, the tasks of mourning are nearing completion.

Although the psychotherapeutic care provided at our voice center follows a brief therapy model, the design of this study called for professional voice users to participate in assessment at three different points which were tied to the time of their diagnosis. The time that elapsed between the first and second session, and between the second and third session, was extremely variable. Nonetheless, the characteristic responses in the domains of affect, cognition, physical sensation, and behavior were evident in these patients whose grief responses predictably are more complex because of some of the factors known to influence grief resolution. These include the unique nature and meaning of the loss to the individual and the strength of his or her attachment to the lost object, in this case, the voice. Ambivalent feelings about the voice often result in an admixture of guilt and anger over the loss.

A related factor is the role and function that the lost object (the voice) filled for the patient in his or her social system. Secondary losses linked to the primary loss increase the amount of grief work because of profound and omnipresent changes the primary loss has brought to the patient's life. It is axiomatic that people grieve in the same way that they cope with other serious stressors, but grief is also influenced by social and familial conditioning. Past experiences with loss, both in number and in resolution, play an enormous role in predicting the outcome of grief response to the loss of voice in these patients. Patients with concurrent psychological illness or other crises in their lives have a relatively more difficult time coping with their grief, and these patients need to be vigilantly monitored for signs of psychiatric decompensation by any psychological professional involved in their care.

Characteristics of the loss itself also appear to affect these patients as they do patients who grieve for the loss of a loved one. These include what has been described as the *death surround*, that is, the immediate circumstances of the loss, its preventability, and whether it was sudden or gradual in onset.[5] Social support is a critical factor; and when it is inadequate, patients will almost always cope less well. Sociocultural, ethnic, gender, and religious backgrounds affect the expression of grief and also determine the amount of support available to the individual. Attitudes consistent with the internal experience of the patient are the most helpful because the patient then has internalized permission to release the grieving affect and ask for and accept support from others.

Finally, physical health influences healing from the bodily injury to the vocal mechanism, and related grief also induces stress responses and their attendant physiologic challenges. Adequate nutrition, rest, and exercise, as well as the avoidance of central nervous system stimulants and depressants, should be advised. Drug therapy should be reserved for psychological decompensation that meets the criteria for major depression or dangerous levels of anxiety response.[4,5]

GUIDED DRAWING ASSIGNMENTS

This is an introduction to the theoretical bases undergirding the use of drawings as a component of diagnostic assessment. The summary is not intended as a review of the exhaustive literature on art therapy. Instead, it attempts to illustrate the value of one projective tool as adapted to this medically ill special population. To the best of the authors' knowledge, these therapeutic principles and techniques have not been used or investigated for therapy with professional voice users or any similar somatically impaired adult population. Preliminary experience in our center suggests that they are of great value. The observations are presented here in case study format. Selected cases are described in detail to assist readers in understanding the evaluation of and rationale behind the clinical insights and principles espoused in this book and their practical applications. More extensive research is needed to confirm the efficacy of the approaches used and to expand and streamline the therapeutic armamentarium.

Important unconscious psychic content is frequently conveyed in drawings, not only by seriously ill people, but also by psychologically and physically healthy people. When this unconscious content is interpreted, it may provide highly valuable therapeutic insight about the individual who has done the drawing. The use of drawings for this purpose was originally designed for therapy with terminally ill children whose capacity for abstract verbal expression is not fully developed. Kübler-Ross[6(p10)] stated that they were therefore open to the use of symbolic means of communication represented by spontaneous drawings. In addition, drawing is a natural medium for children because of its inherent familiarity to them. Her work has shown that drawings allow for an interplay of information between expressed and repressed areas of the individual psyche.[6-8]

Many of the current theories about interpretation of art evolved from work by psychoanalyst Carl Jung.[9] Jung focused on the importance of symbols as messages from the unconscious. This work was applied to medically ill patients by Susan Bach, whose research demonstrated that unconscious content in drawings can be interpreted psychologically and, through that process, provide information about what is happening in the body.[10] The method of interpretation used in our center is described by Greg Furth. Furth[11] reviews the theories of Jung with regard to the unconscious and its representation in art through images and symbols.

Jung believed that "the psyche is a self-regulating system" and that "there is no balance, no system of self-regulation without opposition."[12(p53-54)] Opposition allows for balance. Jung's theory of compensation is based on opposites, balancing and adjusting of the psyche as necessary as it deals with life. The theory suggests that the unconscious either complements or compensates the conscious, always striving for balance. When the unconscious content in a picture coincides with the conscious world, it is said to be *complementary. Compensation* in a drawing depicts an opposition to the conscious world. The aim of all analytical psychology is to discover what the unconscious is saying and to raise it to the level of consciousness. Symbols from the unconscious act in either compensatory or complementary relationship to the conscious status *at a given moment in time.* Compensatory symbols express neglected areas in an attempt to bring them to the attention of consciousness and promote changes in conscious attitude.[12]

Drawings are projective techniques and are based on the defense mechanism of projection, that is, ascribing to another (or an object or creature) beliefs and/or feelings about the self. Numerous projective tests are used commonly in batteries for psychological assessment. These include Rorschach testing, Thematic Apperception Tests, and structured drawing assignments such as the House-Tree-Person (HTP), or kinetic family drawing (KFD) tasks.[13] The value of these instruments is proportional to the skill of the clinician using them. Clinical predictions based on projective tests are said to be helpful provided they are not accepted as final conclusions about personality, but are constantly tested against information elicited through subsequent inquiry, reaction to therapy, and other behavior of the patient.[13-15] According to Furth,[11] systematic analysis of drawings furthers understanding and awareness of these messages from the unconscious, enhancing development and revealing information about the various parts of an individual's personality, mind, and body.

Therapists who use drawing and other projective techniques must remain particularly aware of the potential for projection of the their own unconscious material and/or unfinished "emotional business" upon the patient's drawings (and other responses). As a result of experiencing and working through our own psychological make-up, mental health professionals are better prepared to help others travel their roads to self-discovery. Furth[11] calls this the *wounded-healer theme*. If the helping professional is able to face his or her "wounds" and work toward healing, he or she is better prepared to help the patient confront personal pain. Experienced psychological professionals are aware that it is impossible to accompany a patient beyond where we ourselves have traveled, and this is apparent in the impasses common to all psychotherapy. It is for this reason that professional ethics demands knowledgeable use of peer consultation and supervision. In drawing interpretation, the therapist must look at the picture, with no preconceived ideas, to "listen to the picture." The picture has no voice, so the therapist lends to it his or her own so that it may speak.

Furth[11] recommends working from three basic premises to understand the language of drawings. First, there is an unconscious, and drawings derive from it. The psychology of the individual is similar to an iceberg, that is, the majority of it lies hidden below the surface. So, the therapist will constantly try to determine what particular symbols may mean *to the patient* and not jump to generalizations regarding their meaning. Second, drawings must be accepted as valid means of communication with the unconscious, conveying its meanings reliably. Reliability in this context means that the content is trustworthy. Validity in a picture means that it shows what it reports to show, for example, undeveloped psychological content. The content of a picture is grounded in the patient's life content; therefore, that perspective can only come from mutual discussion. The third premise is that mind and body are inherently linked, and through this linkage they continually communicate and cooperate.

As therapists gain experience in working with drawings from patients with medical diagnoses, the element of forecast is often noted. Drawings may give insight to future happenings within the external world of the patient and therefore offer solutions to life problems. When patients are seriously or terminally ill, elements of the drawing may correlate with major events along the remainder of the patient's life journey. Therefore, drawings can offer the therapist diagnostic information about psychological and physical conflicts and needs, prognostic information, and information about the patient's death awareness and death conceptualization.

In beginning the process of picture interpretation, it is critical to emphasize that the work is done with the patient, not with the picture. The goal is therapeutic empathy and enhanced communication. There are no acceptable "cookbook" interpretations to a drawing. Patients draw particular symbols which they select from their personal world. They use these to share intimate information about the personal self with the therapist. The therapist must understand the conditions under which the picture is drawn and the developmental level and age of the individual, especially with children. A somewhat systematic approach is then used. Furth states that there is "only one rule for picture interpretation: to know that one does not know."[11(p34)] The analyst should be sensitive to his or her initial impression of a picture and concentrate on the initial feeling. The analyst acts as a researcher, understanding the materials used in the picture, the size of the paper in relationship to the size of the drawing, and the focal points. Attempts to synthesize what has been learned from the individual components and assemble this information into a whole comprise the therapist's task.

Furth's[11] techniques of picture interpretation involve the use of focal points, and these will be enumerated and very briefly described. In viewing and understanding the art produced by the patients in the study, Furth's focal points were used to draw preliminary impressions about the patient's unconscious view of him- or herself and his or her voice at each of three sessions during the therapy process.

Initially, the therapist strives to capture a *spontaneous impression of affect*. This is most accurate when it can be described in one word. The therapist can inquire how the person felt while drawing the picture to assess for congruence between the patient's experience and the therapist's response. *What is odd?* In examining the drawing, the therapist tries to discover items that are peculiar or abnormal representations and incompletions. These are thought to reflect problem areas in the patient's life about which the unconscious knows, but may not yet have been brought out into the open. *Are there barriers?* In analyzing the drawing, notes should be made of where barriers are located. These may be inanimate or living, and one can note who is blocking whom from communicating or being in contact. *What is missing?* It is important to observe what is absent or left out of the picture because the missing elements may be of symbolic significance to the patient. They often represent or symbolize what is absent from the patient's life. Missing individuals are described as signs of conflict. *What is central?* Furth emphasizes that what is drawn in the center of the picture may indicate where the core of the problem lies or what is important to the individual. When scars appear in a picture, they are frequently central and often indicate trauma.[11]

What are the size relationships? The proportion of the elements of a drawing is important; and when things are out of proportion, the therapist needs to discover what the excessively large figures emphasize and what the excessively small figures attempt to devalue. *Are there shape distortions?* When some part of a figure or object is drawn out of proportion, it may symbolically represent problem areas that require concentration and investigation. Shape distortions in self-portraits very frequently reveal somatic conditions. *Are there repeated objects?* Objects may be repeated in drawings; and when this occurs, it is usually useful to count them. Furth and Kübler-Ross note that the number of objects is frequently significant and relates to units of time or events of importance in the past, present, or future.[7,11] The element of repetition is one of the features involved in the forecasting noted in drawings by terminally ill patients, especially children.

What perspective does the artist use in drawing the picture? As the therapist observes the picture, the perspective and its relative consistency are noted. When there are different perspectives within the same drawing, this may relate to inconsistencies within the individual's life. What can be seen as you *carry yourself into the picture?* The therapist attempts to become the objects within the picture in order to see, hear, and feel how they behave and understand their relationship to the picture as a whole. This is similar to a technique of Gestalt dream work in which a patient is asked to become, experience and speak for each element of the dream.

Where is the shading? Objects that are shaded take more time and energy to produce and may reflect obsession with or anxiety about what the shaded object represents symbolically. *Is there edging?* Edging consists of an object or element of the picture which is drawn along the edge of the paper so that it appears to go off the paper and is only partially visible. Furth[11] states that edging is like "hedging;" it is a method of revealing something partially and remaining on the "outer limits." *How does the drawing compare to the surrounding world?* Drawings must be compared to the actual physical world beyond that which is represented in the picture, including country, culture, race, religion, and season of the year. When there are differences between what exists in the actual surrounding world and what is represented in a drawing, the difference is said to be significant in terms of the patient's psychological adjustment.

Encapsulation and extensions? Encapsulation symbolizes enclosure, the need to draw boundaries around the self and set oneself apart. Extensions are devices drawn into the hand or arm of a figure which allow the individual to exert greater control over the environment. *Is anything drawn on the back of the paper?* Locating an object or figure on the back of the main drawing may indicate conflict or separation. According to Furth, *underlining* represents lack of grounding and is a complementary symbol. When every individual in the drawing is underlined except one, the person without the underlining is thought to be most grounded. Notice *erasures* and compare the redrawn work with them. Erasures seem to indicate conflict or reworked areas of what the symbol represents in the patient's life. When the redrawn material is an improvement, the patient may have gained control over a difficult area. When the redrawn material deteriorates, this often seems to have been the case in conscious reality, as well.

Are there words in the drawing? Words added to a drawing capture attention and are most often utilized by patients who fear they may not be understood or may be misinterpreted. *Is there lining across the top of the page?* This indicates "something" psychologically overhead which is frequently a burden to the patient or is fearful. *Transparency* is seeing through a barrier to something within. This is developmentally normal in children. In adolescents and adults, transparency of this type appears to reflect seeing into a taboo area. When *movement* is noted in a picture, it is important to follow the trajectory of movable objects, noting their direction and determining the consequences.

Abstract drawings appear to represent something difficult to understand, or may be used as an avoidance. When patients are asked "What does this remind you of?" or "What does this look like to you?" they frequently will make important associations to problems they were unable to draw realistically. Some symbols have particular archetypal meaning. For example, trees are seen as a life symbol. In examining them, notice whether they are balanced, healthy, and grounded in the earth. Notable markings and wounds on the tree should also be correlated to the age of the patient. Questions about time periods in the person's life which correspond to these markings often reveal significant information being offered by the unconscious. Furth describes the use of the tree symbols as "arbor vitae" (tree of life) in which the therapist divides the tree from its base to its top according to the patient's age and notes the placement of particular markings on the tree.

Butterflies reflect transformational change, metamorphosis. To become a butterfly, a caterpillar passes through a state of dissolution to become a winged creature. This is the archetypal symbol for life, death, and resurrection. Butterflies in drawings often reflect innate knowledge of one's life journey, but an absence of fear. The use of the sun in a picture may symbolize energy and warmth, and rainbows remain universal symbols of hope.[1]

Many theories exist about the possible significance of color, but different theories about color interpretation do not always agree on a specific meaning. Most theorists agree that colors can symbolize certain feelings and moods. The use of a particular color and its placement in a drawing may suggest the importance of a psychological or physical element or an imbalance in the patient's life. Color analysis is only a supplemental aid in understanding drawings and may be misunderstood and misinterpreted very easily. Rather than focusing on the specific meaning of an individual color, it is probably more useful to consider how, where, and in what quantity color is used.[11] One should be certain that the patient has had available a full range of color (crayons, markers, pencils, paints) before ascribing significance to the use of *any* color. It is not uncommon for therapists in the early stages of working with drawings to become concerned about a drawing done all in black only to discover that the creator of the picture had only a black marker available to use!

The interpretations which follow are drawn mainly from the work of Bach and are associated with interpretations in Western culture.[10] Her color interpretations were compiled from drawings of seriously ill patients. Red is associated with issues of vital significance, "burning" problems, surging emotions, or danger. It may reflect acute illness, as well, for example, infection or fever. Pink is a less intense hue of red and may suggest the resolution of a problem or illness just past. The color purple symbolizes royalty, spirituality, or focus of control. Orange is associated with suspenseful situations and a decreasing energy flow. The golden yellow color often selected for representations of the sun may emphasize life-giving energy and things of an intuitive or extremely valued nature.[10]

Bright blue denotes health and the vital flow of life. Dark green is associated with health and ego, and paler, yellower greens with psychological or physical weakness. Dark brown reflects nature and the earth, whereas pale brown may denote decay or a struggle to overcome destructive forces. Black may symbolize the unknown and, when used for shading, dark thoughts, threats, or fears. White, according to several authors, is the absence of color and may indicate repressed feelings, purity, or life's completion. Color merely amplifies what the remainder of the picture is attempting to say.[10]

Many expressive arts therapists place great importance on the use of quadrant assessment in drawing interpretation, ascribing specific meanings to each of these quadrants. In Furth's research, the validity and reliability of this form of interpretation was not proven and those trained by him have absorbed his caution in its use. Therapists who are interested in additional data on this subject are referred to Bolander,[14] Bach,[10] Kübler-Ross,[7] Jung,[9] and Jolles.[15]

PSYCHOLOGICAL CONSEQUENCES OF PERCEIVED VOICE LOSS IN PROFESSIONAL VOICE USERS: A RESEARCH STUDY

The pilot study conducted was designed to determine the potential value of in-depth research on the psychological consequences of perceived voice loss in professional voice users. Results are reviewed here in case study fashion, and samples of the instruments are included in Appendix I. Selected cases are described in detail to assist the reader in absorbing the rationale behind our approach and its practical application.

Psychological evaluation of study participants, including relevant psychiatric and psychosocial history, current mental status, specific attention to current and cumulative psychological stressors (especially losses), and significant changes in lifestyle was performed. Coping responses to perceived voice impairment in the selected population were identified and revealed signs and symptoms of grief response in the interviews, self-report responses, and assigned drawings. The following case studies represent a small sample of the patients who agreed to participate in the pilot study. Common psychological characteristics of these individuals including their cognitive, affective, and behavioral presentation relative to their phase of vocal injury are described. As was expected, these phases often overlapped and recurred, and the emotional responses were not entirely linear.

PATIENT EXAMPLES

Case I

This patient was in his mid-40s and was employed as a professor, singer, and choral conductor. He also performed regularly and delivered seminars and workshops nationally. Five weeks prior to his evaluation at our voice center, he had noted sudden onset of hoarseness and loss of his upper range. He was seen by a variety of other voice professionals, but an accurate diagnosis was not established. His initial strobovideolaryngoscopic examination revealed prior vocal fold hemorrhage with a subsequent vocal fold mass. At the first session, items in all domains of the grief inventory were strongly endorsed. He was experiencing distorted cognitions including preoccupation, auditory delusions of the lost voice, confusion, disbelief, and shock. He reported severe insomnia. His affect was anxious, sad, and somewhat angry. He reported significant difficulty with feelings of helplessness and guilt. Anergia and generalized fatigue were present. During the interview, his responses to the personal meaning question included such statements as, "This is who I am, always, since I was 5 years old; it's all I do well." Themes included guilt ("abusing my gift and being punished"), shock ("that I could get hurt"), and impulsiveness (moving for closure in situations because of uncomfortable anxiety even when cognitively aware that such closure was premature). The patient described his most reliable coping responses as "goal setting" and "being a leader." These customary responses were not helpful in the face of the injury. "I identify the problem after precise assessment; fix it objectively; and get on with life, but it isn't working with this; I feel vulnerable and helpless."

The self-portrait produced at the first session was a pen drawing of a disembodied face (Fig 17-1). The eyes were cast upward with a pleading expression, and the brow was creased. The face contained no nose and sealed lips, allowing neither an airway nor communication. The representation in response to the request "Draw your voice." was abstract, represented by a negative sine wave with points plotted for past, present, and future (Fig 17-2). Prior to diagnosis, this patient's loss history had included only a severe lower back problem 1 year prior to the onset of his voice symptoms. He himself characterized the voice loss as "devastating, as my entire careers revolves around and employs my voice."

Six months later, the patient had undergone vocal fold surgery and ongoing voice therapy. He reported that the prognosis for return of normal voice was excellent. In the interim, he had experienced a divorce with its consequent secondary losses, and these items were endorsed as extremely negative on the modification of the Holmes and Rahe scale.[13] He had also lost some traditional sources of psychosocial support. He described his coping repertoire as including exercise, positive thoughts, daily prayer, and meditation, as well as "people who *do* care." At 6 months postdiagnosis, the grief inventory reflected endorsement of fewer items in the domain of physical sensations, but still in-

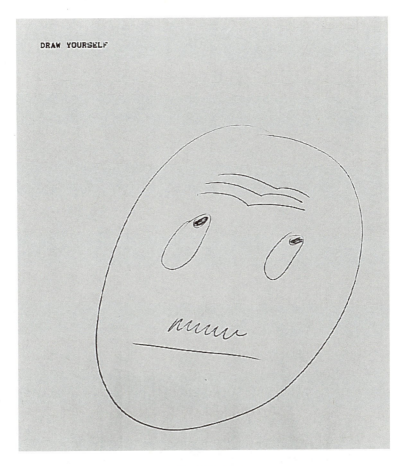

FIGURE 17-1

cluded some anergia, gasping, hollowness in the "center," and depersonalization. This instrument was designed by the authors, based on
the work of Worden.[4] Cognition was improving, but confusion and
preoccupation with the voice were still reported. Every item in the affect domain was endorsed except self-reproach. Behavior was still significantly affected with sleep and appetite disturbance, social withdrawal, sighing, crying, and dreams of the lost voice reported.

During the interview, this singer reported that he was "doing better" with the effects of the vocal injury on his level of physical experience, but that he was uncertain how well he was reacting and still had
significant anxiety about reinjury. When asked to interpret the meaning
of the impact of the voice injury in his life context, he reported he was

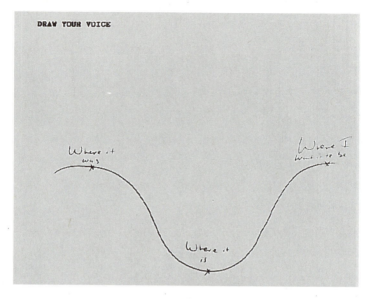

FIGURE 17-2

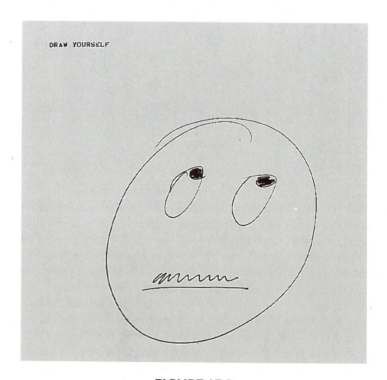

FIGURE 17-3

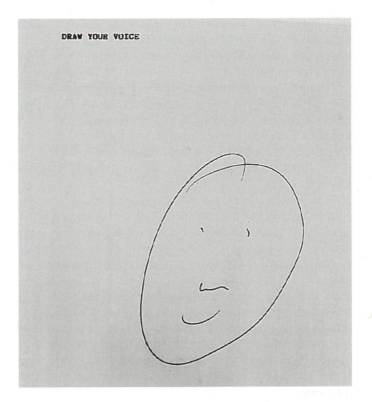

FIGURE 17-4

still struggling with its message, especially since it was imbedded in such a period of personal relationship turmoil. His self-portrait was similar to that produced at the first session, but it was done in blue (Fig 17-3). The gaze was still upcast, and there was still no nose. However, the mouth was parted slightly. The patient's representation of the voice was now similar to his self-portrait, but with eyes focused, a nose, and a slight smile (Fig 17-4). The patient had not been discharged from active treatment at the conclusion of the pilot study.

Case 2

Case 2 involved a 36-year-old classical singer for whom church solo work, oratorio, recital, and opera were her primary performance opportunities, on a part-time basis. She was also an actor and director in community and school theater. She noted the onset of hoarseness after a particularly strenuous rehearsal while performing in another city. She was seen emergently by an otolaryngologist there who diagnosed a vocal fold mass but no acute hemorrhage. She was able to complete the performance, but returned with persistent hoarseness. On strobovideolaryngoscopic examination at our voice center, she was noted to have a superior laryngeal nerve paresis, significant gastroesophageal reflux laryngitis, and bilateral vocal fold masses. She engaged in a period of intensive voice therapy and went on to surgical excision. In the immediate postoperative period, she developed an upper respiratory infection with prolonged and severe coughing that led to a left vocal fold tear and scar formation. Sequential steroid injection into the vocal fold was performed.

At the first session, there was strong endorsement of three domains of the grief inventory, but the only cognitive item endorsed was disbelief. The strongest of these sets was in the domain of affect where the typical early responses to loss were noted: sadness, anger, shock, numbness, and anxiety. She reported periods of derealization and hyperarousal, as well as significant social withdrawal. This patient had experienced numerous prior losses with frequent moves and loss of her support network and musical identity. At the time of her injury, she felt a severe lack of social support. Her coping repertoire included an outward focus on her family, positive activities, meditation, and prayer. The patient felt sustained by a belief that she was "given the gift of strength and the ability to carry on." She reported that she tended to use anger as a defense for anxiety and depression and to be plagued by negative internal dialogue.

At the first session, her self-portrait consisted of a 1 cm stick figure drawn in pencil in the very center of the page (Fig 17-5). This figure was faceless and had neither hands nor feet. The patient reported extreme discomfort with the drawing task and stated that she "came from a family of artists." This theme was to recur. Her drawing of her voice was also a pencil sketch of an empty, centered oval with the edges shaded and extending outward (Fig 17-6). Both the figure and the rays slanted significantly to the left of the page. In the loss history, she listed multiple moves with inherent loss of dear friends and patterns of interaction with family, as well as the severing of musical contacts, the loss of the support system as a whole, and loss of sense of identity. There had also been the death of a great aunt and an altercation with her in-laws in which she felt a sense of estrangement from her spouse. In addition, she described the loss of an opportunity to sing a role which was "almost guaranteed" as quite traumatic, and this caused her to stop singing completely for a 3-month period.

The second session occurred 4 months after diagnosis and surgery. The grief inventory at that time revealed that derealization and hyper-

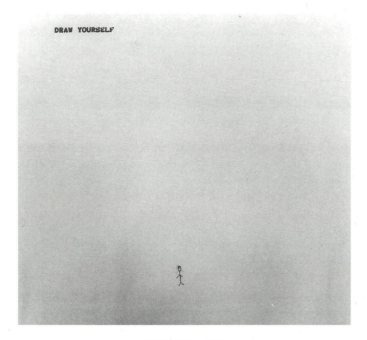

FIGURE 17-5

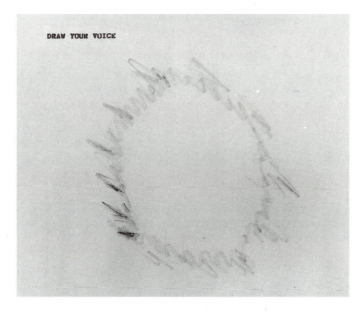

FIGURE 17-6

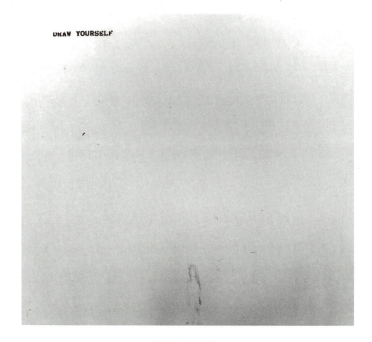

FIGURE 17-7

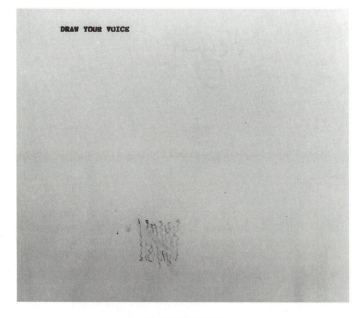

FIGURE 17-8

arousal continued, and there were some auditory delusions of the "lost voice." She described herself as withdrawn, crying, and avoiding all stimuli of her lost voice (people and places). Endorsement was strongest in the affect domain with sadness, anger, self-reproach, anxiety, fatigue, helplessness, and numbness selected. Her coping repertoire at that time consisted of an increase in physical exercise, reading for escape, frequent crying which seemed to release some of the ache, and a personally designed refrain "breaking down the unmanageable into grains of sand." At the second session, she described loss of support and contact from her spouse who was being required to travel frequently by his business and who was emotionally drained by the stresses of his job.

Replies to the personal meaning questions in the interview revealed that the patient derived from a family of successful performing artists. She felt that she never measured up to their abilities and was "probably afraid to try and fail and never gave it my full effort." At the time of her injury, she had just returned from a successful summer performing in Europe and had begun to accrue soloist roles. She described this as "just beginning to think of myself as a real singer." Her drawings at that time included a self-portrait with a slightly larger pencil figure, no longer a stick figure (Fig 17-7). At that time, it possessed hair, limbs, and feet, but no face, hands, or trunk. The back was slightly shaded, and the figure continued to face obliquely to the left. Her drawing of her voice consisted of nine wavering lines, each 1 cm in length (Fig 17-8). The pencil drawing was marred by erasure slashes obliquely from the upper left to the lower right which distorted and partially eliminated the lines. The patient had not been discharged from active treatment at the completion of the pilot phase.

Case 3

This professional business speaker and lay minister was in his late 40s. He reported persistent hoarseness for a 6-month period prior to evaluation at the voice center. Initial strobovideolaryngoscopic examination revealed the presence of bilateral vocal fold masses and very significant gastroesophageal reflux laryngitis. Significant muscular tension dysphonia in both the singing and speaking voice were present. At the first session, the patient endorsed items on all four domains of the grief inventory, most significantly in the area of affect (guilt, self-reproach, anxiety, shock, and sadness). He was also troubled by sleep disturbance and social withdrawal. He reported derealization and preoccupation with the lost voice, as well as confusion and hyperarousal to stimuli. During the interview, with regard to the personal meaning of this injury, the patient reported that he had had a strong history of prior heavy alcohol intake and smoking, but had successfully halted both of these after making a serious, personal religious commitment. He expressed significant fear that his hoarseness reflected the presence of laryngeal cancer. The patient's interpretation of the meaning of his injury was, "another lesson, another test of will and faith." He was determined to *"beat* the problem" and the labile emotions that surrounded it. He reported that past increases in anxiety had always prompted a response of excessive control, bargaining, and self-sacrifice. His coping repertoire included logic and the development of clear goals and commitments. He described himself as able to communicate his personal needs to his family and very supported by prayer and the ability to refocus and reframe events to the positive. A sloganlike summary of that attitude consisted of the phrase, "transcending the circumstance in attitude and action." The patient had listed instances of loss at the first session including loss of relationships with significant people and wandering away from his relationship with God. In addition, he cited the loss of his clear voice.

Art from the first session consisted of a self-portrait revealing a round, concentric circle figure of his head, body core, and lower limbs (Fig 17-9). No feet, arms, or face were included. The neck was drawn as a single spindle extending from the area of the neck to mid-face. One circle had a very noticeable break as it crossed the neck on the right side of the page. It was unclear whether this was a front or a rear view of the patient. His drawing of his voice consisted of words written in stylistic script. The word *smooth* was highly angulated to the right of the page and compressed. *Soothe* was spelled without the final e and was more upright.

The patient was treated with voice therapy, but the vocal fold masses persisted. The second session was conducted approximately 3 months postoperatively. At that time, endorsement in all three domains was again present. Significant in the domain of affect was the absence of guilt, but the addition of helplessness. Physical symptoms included continued hyperarousal to sensory stimuli and derealization. There were shifts in all domains toward anergia, withdrawal, and the expression of sorrow. The patient's coping repertoire at that time consisted of prayer and Bible study along with recreational reading and billiards. He felt that he had reestablished his goals, but was rethinking his approaches to his world of work. Both clear goal setting and creativity were highly valued response criteria for this man. His loss history described loss of "personal voice" and a loss of professional speaking engagements. Because professional speaking was this patient's primary

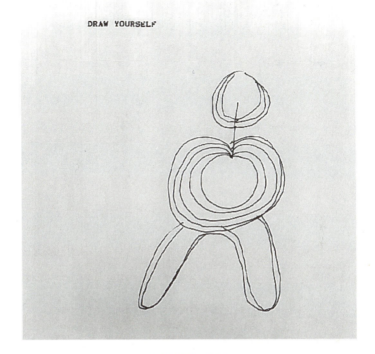

DRAW YOURSELF

FIGURE 17-9

occupation, there were significant effects on his financial status, as well as his occupational identity. Art at the second session included a self-portrait stick figure with three circles: one for the head, one for the thorax, and one for the abdomen and pelvis (Fig 17-10). This was rendered in ball-point ink. The figure's legs and arms were outstretched, with a broad base of support. There were no feet or hands, no face, and no neck. A stick pierced the figure from abdomen to the area where the mouth would customarily be drawn. His portrayal of the voice consisted of a wavering ink line with a vector to the left (Fig 17-11). The arrow was blunted, and the patient commented that this reflected a change in his approach to life demands from "sharp and incisive to widespread but persistent force." Figures 17-12 and 17-13 were produced prior to a clinical session. The patient was referred to the author (DCR) because of his speech pathologist's concerns about his mood. The patient was asked to draw a self-portrait and to draw his voice on the evening prior to his psychotherapeutic session. The self-portrait is devoid of facial

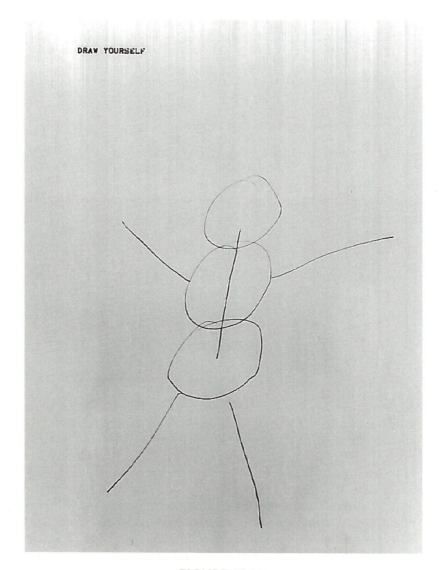

DRAW YOURSELF

FIGURE 17-10

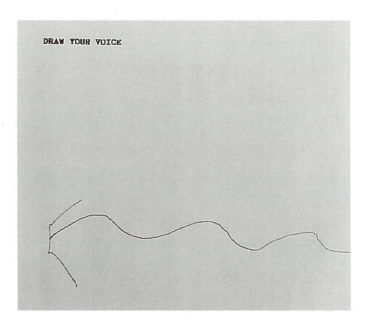

FIGURE 17-11

features with the exception of a mouth. The mouth is drawn as a sine wave, with an upward tilt to the mouth surrounding the term "life" and a downward curve to the mouth covering the word "voice." The patient drew the neck region with a midline division. He described the figure as representing the oscillating, labile emotional reactions he was then experiencing. Using terminology characteristic for splitting, he stated, "On the one hand, my life focus has never been healthier: my personal and spiritual priorities are straight. On the other hand, my voice quality rose only to decline. I am so very fearful that it will continue on this downward course." Interestingly, the lower limbs of the pictured figure are not grounded, and the patient commented that he experienced his professional, voice-dependent, future as "up in the air." The drawing of his voice reflected the initial, gradual upward progression of his vocal quality. With significant support and encouragement during the therapy session, he expressed fear about the oscillations evident in the middle section of the diagram. "There have been so many ups and downs, I fear that the instability and roller coaster will lead to a plummet and that I will also fall and fail." The patient had not been discharged from active treatment by the pilot's closing date.

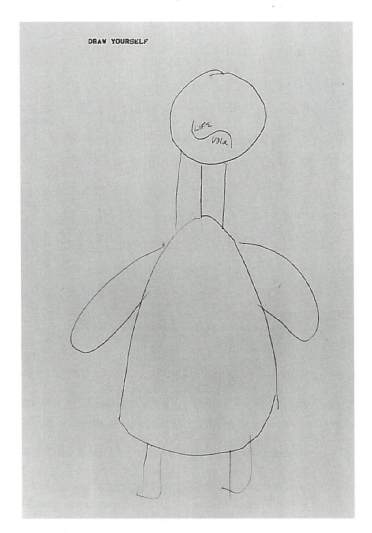

FIGURE 17-12

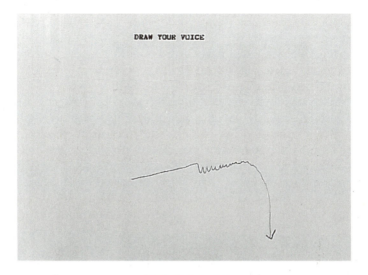

FIGURE 17-13

Case 4

This 17-year-old high school student noted the onset of vocal difficulty 1 year prior to her evaluation at the voice center. In spite of her youth, she was extremely talented and was actively planning a professional singing career after graduation. The patient had been performing actively since the age of 6. During that time, she had been treated for allergy and gastroesophageal reflux laryngitis, but noted continued trouble with intonation, endurance, and the highest notes in her range. She also played a wind instrument on a regular basis. At the time of her evaluation at the center, diagnoses of ARIAS (a form of asthma), muscular tension dysphonia, improper singing technique, gastroesophageal reflux laryngitis, and bilateral vocal fold masses, at least one a probable post-hemorrhagic cyst, were made.

At the first session, she endorsed items in all four domains, and the primary affect was one of shock and numbness with some associated guilt. Derealization and preoccupation with the lost voice were reported (using exclamation points). Her behaviors included distractibility and "sorrow," both maladaptive in her role as a high school student. Her coping repertoire consisted of talking to and listening to others (especially peers with similar problems). She described locking herself in her room and crying to herself, becoming very moody, and praying. At the first session, this patient cited the loss of her boyfriend and loss of her voice with effects on her ability to try out for school plays, temporary loss of "my gift," and the loss of her familiar school and the associated peer group.

During the interview, there were several responses to the question about personal meaning: "If my voice is gone, I am gone." "This is teaching me to appreciate my gift . . . It was a sin to have wasted it." "You can't change what happened in the past. Just cope and keep going." These reflected the fact that performing had become her identity with both her peers and her parents, and she was attempting to find ways to reframe and refocus the experience. Members of the voice team were concerned about potentially self-injurious or self-destructive behaviors, and it was a concern that the patient could not create an image of herself in the future without "her" voice. At the same time, she stated, "I just want to be a kid again . . . This is the cost of showing off."

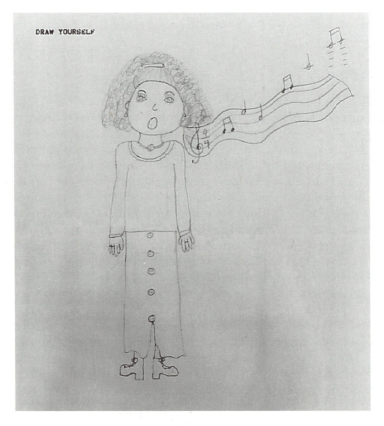

FIGURE 17-14

Art produced at the first session included a self-portrait which consisted of a realistic pencil sketch of a young girl with no secondary sex characteristics (Fig 17-14). The shoulders were held very high. The mouth was open, and the tongue was pulled far back in the mouth. A musical staff extended upward and away from the mouth, and it reached above high C. Her representation of the voice was also a pencil sketch (Fig 17-15). The page was divided vertically and labeled "before operation" and "after operation." On the "before" side of the

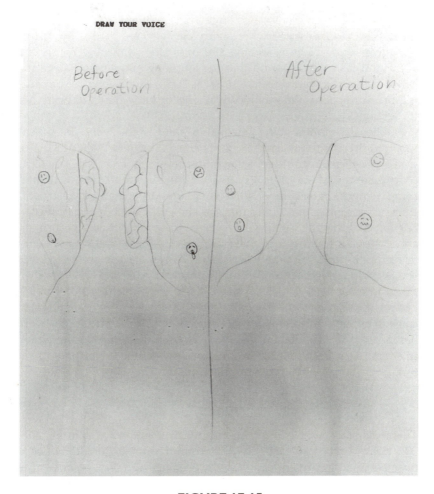

FIGURE 17-15

page, the patient drew what she described as her vocal folds which demonstrate granular edges with bilateral protuberances (Fig 17-15). The vocal folds contained small, round faces representing "angry, queasy, terrified, and sad." In the area of the picture labeled "after operation," the vocal fold edges are calm and smooth, and the inset faces reflect "happiness, scrutiny (consisting of an artificially pronounced smiling face), singing (with a frightened look in the eyes), and a squeezed mouth with downcast eyes." The images are more positive, but still reflect ambivalence.

At the second session, the patient preferred not to complete the self-report materials, nor would she draw. During the interview, she described her coping repertoire as including a very supportive instrumental music teacher who encouraged her to "blare" her wind instrument, beat on drums, and write poetry. She also reported sleep disturbance consisting of hypersomnia and difficulty awakening for school. She enthusiastically reported that her speaking and singing voice felt better at the voice center where she was "safe," but she was experiencing pressure because it was inconvenient for her parents to bring her for sessions.

In her description of the personal meaning of the event, the patient reported that she felt that she "didn't belong anywhere right now." She was experiencing significant polarization between parental advice to be practical and prepare to be a teacher and the desire to "go for it" and pursue a performing career. The patient experienced emotional support from her parents around pursuits consistent with a more practical goal. She felt that they had given up on their image of her as a performer, and she found it difficult to sustain it on her own. Asked why she preferred not to work with the self-report and art materials, she stated that she felt "ripped in two" and didn't want to appear "too crazy." When asked to close her eyes and describe her internal picture of her voice, her posture loosened; facial muscle tone softened, and a small smile came to her lips. "It's there. It's all better, and it's free and supple" were her descriptors. The patient had not yet been discharged from active treatment, and additional voice therapy was planned. Her parents refused further psychotherapeutic intervention.

Case 5

This male singer, songwriter, and jazz instrumentalist was in his late-30s. He had received classical vocal training in college. He owned a business and performed mostly in the evenings and on weekends. The patient presented to the voice center with a 3-week duration of sudden-onset, total aphonia after being struck in the chin and anterior neck during a basketball game. This had been treated with voice rest, and his speaking voice gradually improved. At the time of his evaluation, his singing voice continued to have restriction of range and diminished projection, especially in the lowest and highest registers. Strobovideo-laryngoscopic examination and imaging studies revealed no evidence of laryngeal fracture or arytenoid dislocation. Superior laryngeal nerve paresis and evidence of a resolved vocal fold hemorrhage, as well as significant muscular tension dysphonia, were present. The patient also complained of hyperacusis in the right ear, but an audiogram revealed normal pure-tone and high-frequency thresholds and speech discrimination. At the first session, the patient endorsed items in all four domains of the grief inventory; these were most prevalent in the domain of affect which was mixed, but included endorsement of a significant number of helplessness items. He also described derealization and some social withdrawal, as well as irritability and impact on his marital relationship.

His prior loss history had included loss of the family business, frequent family relocations, loss of significant relationships, and the loss of the "easy qualities" of his early marriage. His coping repertoire included "making music" (instrumental), social contact with others, and the ability to use previously learned relaxation skills. However, he was also engaging in excessive exercise and alcohol consumption. Because of the potentially deleterious effects of these choices, more adaptive strategies were suggested by the author at the first session, including journalizing. The patient then journalized in the form of stream-of-consciousness letters which were sent to the therapist and revealed a clear progression through the cognitive, affective, physical, and behavioral manifestations of grief reaction.

During the interview, the patient's description of the personal meaning of the event included: "My voice was my ticket out of the family farm to college as a music major where I discovered my instrument." The voice was "the intimate and personal part of my self." His self-concept at that time was otherwise poor, and his physical attractiveness did not fit with his sense of self. He described himself as a perfectionistic person for whom his voice was his "best accomplishment." He described obsessive fears of trying to achieve a positive self-definition without his voice. The patient struggled with restrained tears throughout the interview and was able to respond to an intervention from the therapist about releasing his breath. This led to a tearful catharsis of grief and loss.

Art from the first session was produced over 2 days. His self-portrait consisted of a blue electric guitar surrounded by the names of performers whom he admired (Plate 17-1). The guitar itself screams

"Help" in red block letters which stream outward. Ghosted behind are a series of wispy, black shapes with geometric forms. The representations of his voice occurred at three separate times after the initial interview (Plate 17-2). The first consists of a full-page background drawn in black with flecks of blue. A central orange question mark nearly fills the page. Several hours later, after continuing the cathartic experience with private tears, the voice was represented by a black spiral containing a central white circle and black dots and dashes (Plate 17-3). This was captioned, "at the end of a long tunnel." By the next morning, the voice was drawn as a red door into a purple room and included the caption, "Door opening into the red-brown room, the room being my voice, I felt myself entering the room." A selection of the quotes from this patient's journal follows. These were excerpted from letters sent to the therapist between the first and second sessions.

> Where has your music gone? Voice is a puzzle, and the outside pieces are put back together . . . I'm putting the middle together piece by piece. The rehab process is not going to be as fast as I want it to . . . When I went back to singing classically, I had this feeling: scared and consumed. The voice (to me) is a very large mysterious psychological entity. (Talking about a speaker blast) "Worried about your voice are you?" God said, "What do you think about deafness?"! It's neat how writing stuff out puts it in perspective.

Two months later at the second session, most of the items endorsed on the grief inventory were from the affect scale (sadness, anger, guilt, helplessness, numbness, and yearning) Some derealization and preoccupation were endorsed on the physical and cognitive scales. The most prominent behaviors are reflective of persistent, mild depression (sleep and appetite disturbance). The coping repertoire being utilized at that time included partying (with significant alcohol intake), playing music, and exercise. The cognitive ability to reframe himself as a whole versus himself as a singer was only intermittently available to him.

Art from that session included a self-portrait which consisted of a page divided in two (Plate 17-4). On the upper portion is a black figure with lips tight, no neck, eyes and mouth fearful, with motion artifact around the shoulders and a caption: "Whatever happens." The lower section of the picture is an arm at the biceps, drawn in blue, and extending to a digitless hand labeled, "It's supposed to be a fist . . . determined to do it!" The drawing of the patient's voice from that session is also divided into two sections (Plate 17-5). In the upper portion of the drawing is a blue jigsaw puzzle; in the lower section, a small question mark in a large white field. This contains the label, "I like the puzzel (sic) better."

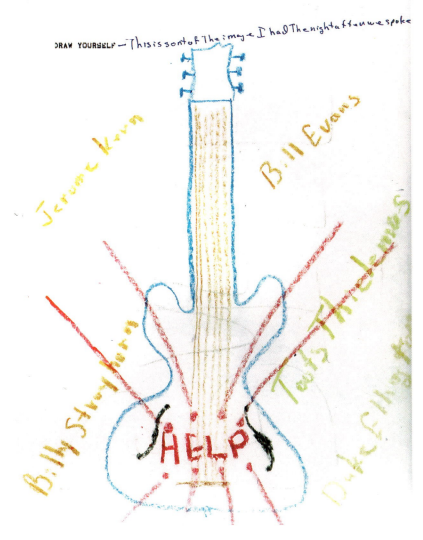

PLATE 17-1

215

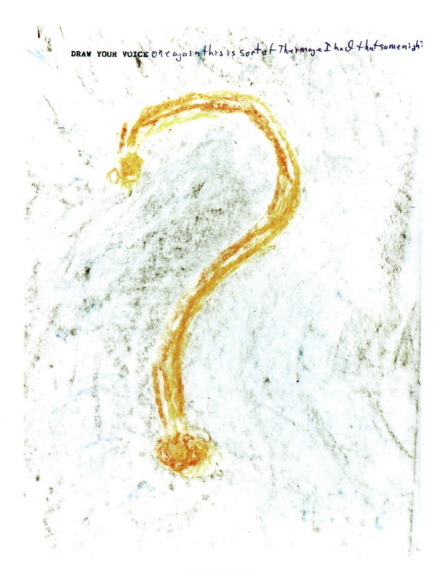

DRAW YOUR VOICE once again this is sort of Thermage I had that same night

PLATE 17-2

216

Images of My Voice

8/3 | 0 8/30 % when we talk - on phone

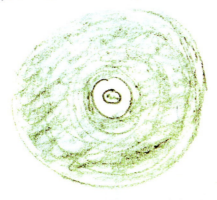

At the end of a long tunnel

7/2

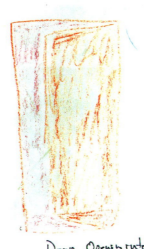

Door Opening into that brown Room/door was opening

the Room being
my Voice
I felt myself
entering the room

PLATE 17-3

This is after Making Copies of types for Karate

I see myself in 2 ways

DRAW YOURSELF

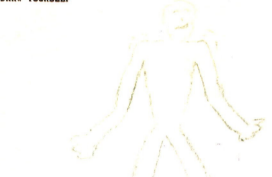

shrugging my Shoulders (whatever happens happens

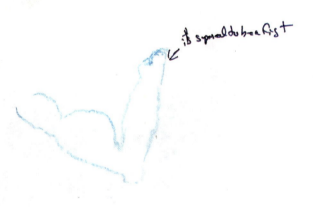

it should be a fist

Determined to do it

PLATE 17-4

I see my voice in ways also

DRAW YOUR VOICE

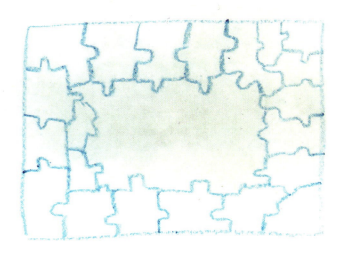

as a puzzel

as a question Mark   I like the puzzel Better!

PLATE 17-5

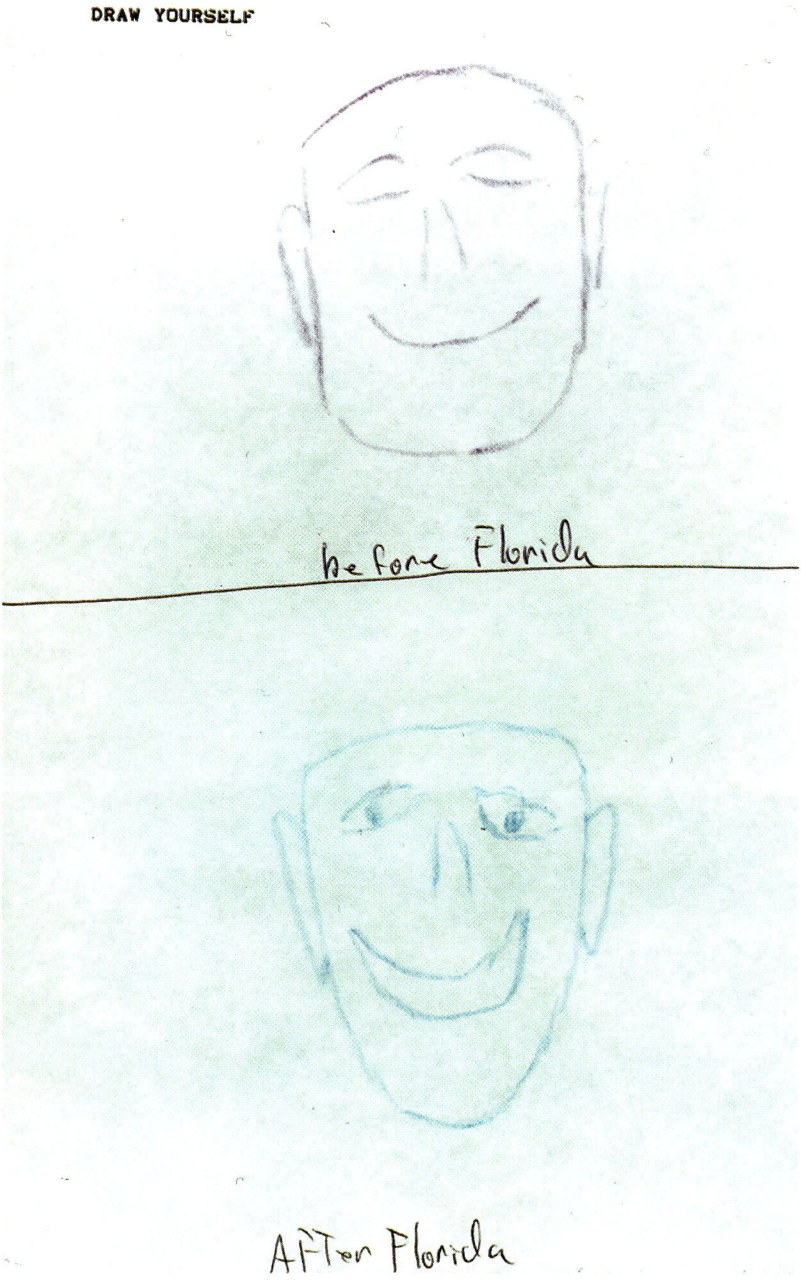

DRAW YOURSELF

before Florida

After Florida

PLATE 17-6

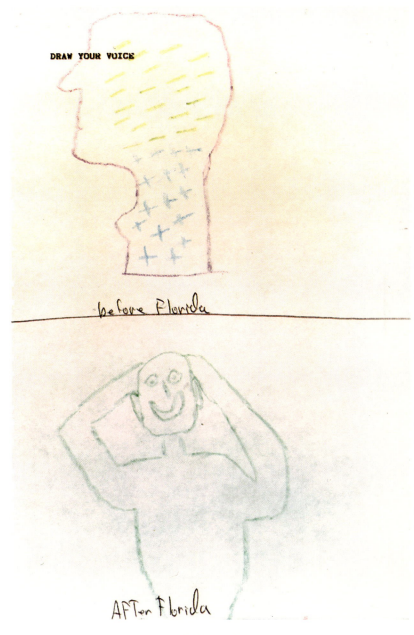

PLATE 17-7

DRAW YOURSELF (USE A NEW BOX OF CRAYONS SO THAT
YOU HAVE ALL COLORS FROM WHICH TO CHOOSE.

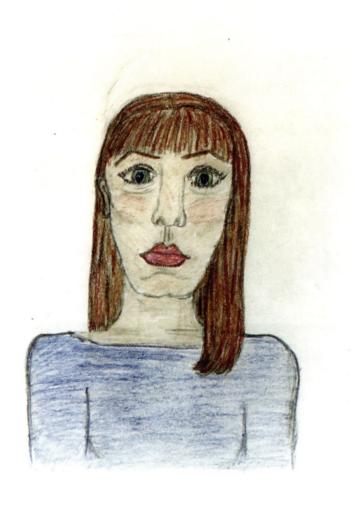

PLATE 17-8

DRAW YOUR VOICE (SAME INSTRUCTIONS AS PRIOR PAGE)

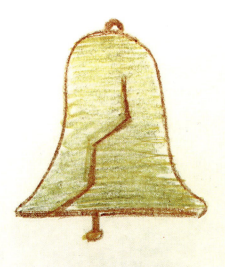

PLATE 17-9

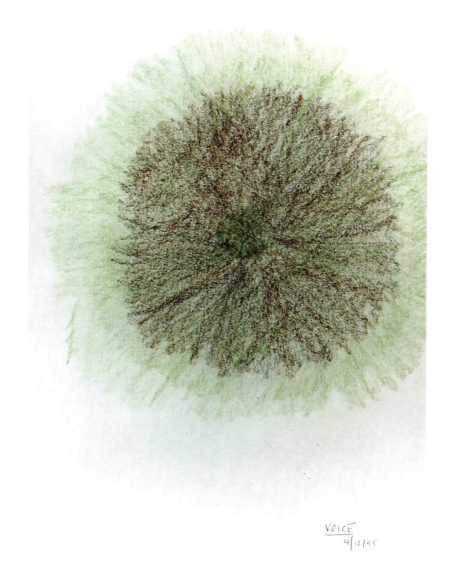

VOICE
4/12/95

PLATE 17-10

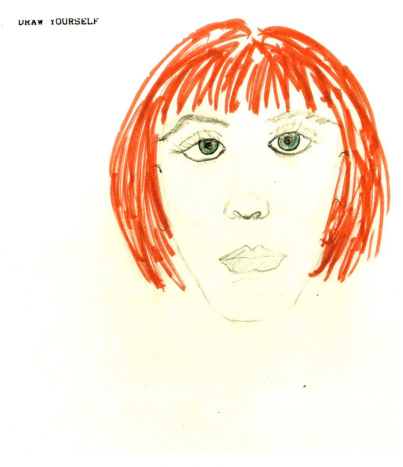

PLATE 17-11

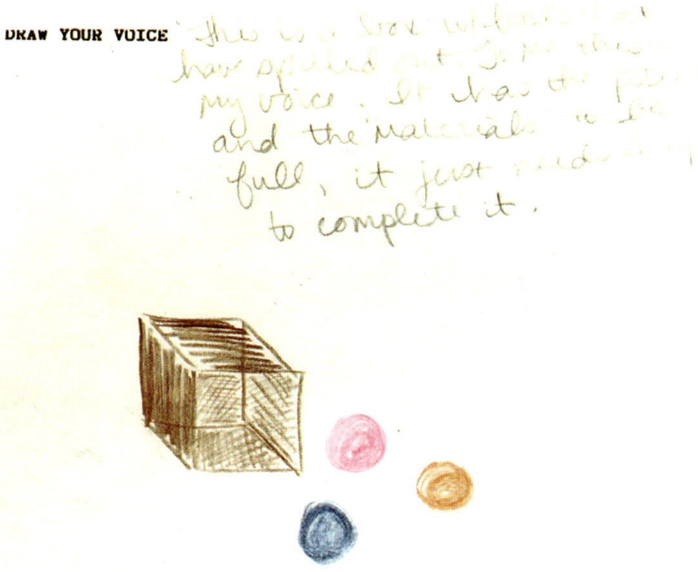

*this is a box w/because I
have spilled out. Is it is there
my voice. It has the pieces
and the materials in it
full, it just needing
to complete it.*

PLATE 17-12

226

During the interview, the patient's description of the personal meaning of his struggle with his voice included the statements, "I had been aloof and arrogant about my vocal abilities and I took them for granted, now I am humbled." He described himself as historically intolerant of "himself with a flaw." One component of the personal meaning of the event and its effects on him was a beginning affirmation of his musicianship in general. He remained uncertain about the return of his voice, and he had begun to struggle with personal feelings about his voice therapist. His internal dialogue consisted of a refrain, "Rework your support." According to the patient, this consisted of physical, vocal, and psychological support.

Quotes from that period of time, including a poem, follow:

I'm not letting go.
I'm holding the voice like old.
No vibrato feel.

Have to connect it
support it, and
let it go free.

Staying in touch with the music is the most important thing now. My easiest avenue has been taken away, but you can't play chords with the voice . . . I feel really strange today . . . innocence or helplessness almost taking over. I feel super-aware, and I know from my past that the most painful things ended up to be the most helpful. If that's the case, I should be benefitting. . . . Self, I want you to come back. Self, I want you back. I really miss my old self. This emotional instability is starting to annoy me, but it is positive because it will motivate me to get back to work. . . . How do I feel about having people help me? I never needed help before. Now I feel inferior *and* a strong sort of gratitude. Thanks for giving me an environment I can work in, or for helping me find me.

After telling a story about working on the business partnership and having a flashback of his original injury,

When I was trying to sing today, the image of the new agreement and the basketball game came into view . . . I tried to sing some high notes, feeling my throat and the day I got injured kept coming back into my mind.

I saw this little image that all I need to do to sing is relax, use my non-manipulated voice, and little by little the range will come back. This is so hard for me! It's in my nature to be overthorough and strive for perfection. That's how I got where I was before. I was given a nice voice, but I worked really hard with it. Now I want to hear myself sing "Refiner's fire" and the "Libera Me" again. . . . I cry in church. I think you're right about my tears and voice being connected. I get this feeling of holding back and preventing my larynx from moving to sing the high notes. . . . One thing is for sure, I will be a fine singer again, and more important, I will be a singer who is a musician! A singer who is a musician is a whole different story than a singer who is a singer. I need, being a musician who has a voice as an instrument. . . . More tears, but happy tears, maybe color in the top comes from happy?! . . . There is something about the voice. Something about the connection between the voice and the person, a connection you helped me put back together. More tears . . . more room inside . . . take deep breaths into an area that feels less . . . and less . . . tense. . . .

After a joint-session with the voice therapist regarding a technique the psychotherapist and the voice therapist designed together in response to their observation of the patient's struggles with vocal technique and emotional impasse, he wrote:

It's like you said, it helps you get the crap out. At the time, it sort of reminded me of puking, but it is a great image to get the bad stuff out!

The patient, knowing the purposes of the research study, provided the following "Rules for Rehabilitation."

1. Stay rested. You have to organize your life so you can stay fresh. Rehabilitation takes a fresh, awake mind and body. I'm sure you can remember having days in the past when you felt good and could do anything you wanted. You have to try to make all your days of rehabilitation like that. What you are doing is hard, and you are unexperienced (sic) at it. It is new. If the people you are working with say you can do it, then you can. It's just a matter of time. How much time depends on how well you can organize your life so you are fresh.
2. You have to rehabilitate yourself. Others will help you, but you have to do the work yourself.
3. Stay relaxed but aware. Learn to balance being aware and overly self-aware. You have to have a sense of self-actualization. You have a task to perform and you can do it. Look at it, analyze it, and conquer it. You will win one step at a time. You have to put your trust in the people you are working with. You are too involved to see the big picture. Just stay with the program.
4. Try to stay ahead of your work. This will reduce stress. The more organized you are about yourself, the faster you will accomplish this task.
5. You are the most important person in your life. Invest this time in yourself. Do it coldly, objectively, and unemotionally if you can.

6. Trauma is very emotional. Try to look at what you have to do objectively without emotion. Work at it as an organizational task. Then you will feel the positive emotions of your progress.
7. The most important thing is to feel like yourself. I believe if you can feel like your old self, then the rehabilitation process will be a lot easier. Remember, organization is self-care, self-care is rest, rest leads to relaxation. A rested, relaxed person can accomplish a lot in a short period of time. This is what you want to do.

The third session was conducted 6 months after the patient's initial evaluation at the center. The grief inventory at that time included a change in domain weighting to the physical. The endorsed items included some derealization and depersonalization along with profound fatigue. The second most significant domain included behaviors, which still included crying, preoccupation with the voice, and sleep disturbance. Coping behaviors at that session revealed balanced exercise, music-making, and the use of hypnosis and massage. The patient reported very little alcohol consumption. Spirituality had taken on a greater support role for him.

The art task at that time included a self-portrait which was again divided into sections (Plate 17-6). These were labeled: before Florida and after Florida. The "before Florida" image was of a purple face with eyes closed and a tight-lipped smile. The "after Florida" representation was a face drawn in blue with a wide smile and eyes open. Also noted was the size distortion between the right and left ears, and the patient continued to complain of hyperacusis on the right. His drawing of the voice again consisted of images "before and after Florida" (Plate 17-7). In the "before" image, a purple profile with green minus signs in the area of the head and to the level of the chin but with blue plus signs in the area of the neck were apparent. The thyroid cartilage was especially prominent. In the "after" image, the upper body was drawn in green to the waist. Arms were folded behind the head. Eyes were open, and there was a wide smile.

During the interview, the patient reported less obsessive thinking and could take pleasure in the consistent psychological benefits of "working through his personal areas of unfinished business." He also described the balance of his "logs" (music and relationships) as more stable. Asked to describe the personal meaning of the events in one sentence, he said, "Music is a gift to be nurtured and groomed." His trips to the voice center for vocal rehabilitation from his home and business in another city were "time out of time" for his voice and for himself.

Following is a selection from quotes derived from letters which continued to arrive between the second and third sessions.

It bothered me that I was so emotionally vulnerable about singing. . . . no one likes to be humiliated. I believe the emotions I feel are just part of the process . . . . You have the voice on one hand and the body on the other, the better shape you get your body into, the faster your voice will heal. . . . I feel really in control of my life, work and my marriage. Maybe this whole experience has enabled me to learn how to cope with things that are difficult. . . . It seems that the emotional highs and lows have stopped. I feel plain and grounded. I feel at peace with myself. I can't remember when I last felt that. . . . Sometimes I think I'm afraid of the real me, then I avoid him chemically. I do have trouble disconnecting my emotions with serious music. I'm just a human being trying to make his voice sound perfect. I think this awareness is good. It is probably my way of opening up and letting the voice reenter my body.

This patient was discharged from active treatment, but continued to journalize intermittently and forward the letters to the therapist. He continued to do well.

Case 6

This patient was a folk singer in his early 30s who had received classical training and had operatic performance experience. He was an active composer and performer of folk music and accompanied himself on his guitar. He was seen and evaluated at the voice center approximately 2 years after his initial symptoms occurred. They originally consisted of an upper respiratory infection and significant seasonal allergies. Subsequently, he noticed decreased pitch accuracy, "fuzziness," loss of vibrato, loss of "ring," loss of his uppermost notes, and significant vocal fatigue. After strobovideolaryngoscopic examination and additional evaluation by the consultant neurologist, he was diagnosed with myasthenia gravis, superior laryngeal nerve paresis, gastroesophageal reflux laryngitis, and a right vocal fold granuloma.

During the first session, the patient endorsed markers in all four domains of the grief inventory. These were most pronounced in the affective domain and least in the cognitive. He was significantly preoccupied with his lost voice, but denied guilt. His loss history included the loss of an intimate relationship, the death of his beloved pet, and the loss of his house due to fire. His coping repertoire included prayer, exercise, walks, warm baths, listening to music, and talking it out with supportive friends.

Art tasks at the first session included a self-portrait drawn representatively in black ink, although all colors of crayons were available

(Fig 17-16). An opening was noted at the crown of the head, and the right arm was atrophic with only four digits drawn in. (He has an overuse injury to the left arm.) There is no neck, and the lips are tightly sealed. His drawing of his voice consists of a tree with open knot hole in the lower third, 3 completed branches, and 2 open and unfinished branches (Fig 17-17). A dog is present and faces away from the tree and the flowers. A swing hangs from the tree, but one of the lines representing the rope is broken and patched together approximately one-third from the bottom.

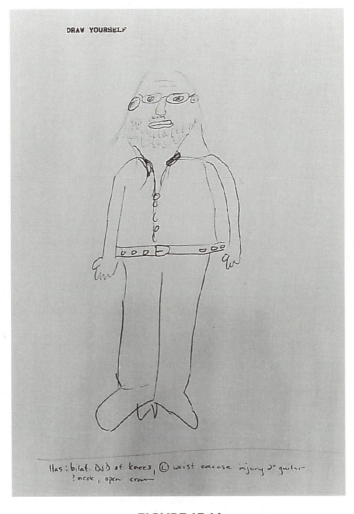

FIGURE 17-16

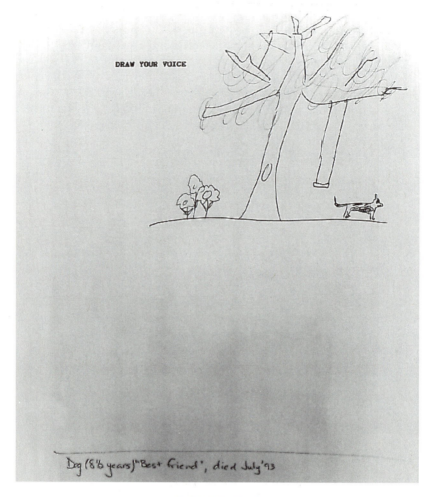

DRAW YOUR VOICE

Dog (8½ years) "Best Friend", died July '93

FIGURE 17-17

During the interview, the patient had several interpretations of the meaning of his voice complaint. They included associations of physical illness to aging and deterioration, the use of his voice to "get smiles" from his family constellation, and negative messages from his "external world" such as, "Singing is a frou-frou career." Questions about the personal meaning of the event also included statements such as, "I've never had anything that broke get fixed in my body." He reported a history of overuse injuries to his arm from guitar playing and from an abusive exercise pattern. He experienced intense support from his spirituality and sought to answer existential/spiritual questions such as, "What is God's intention for me?" and held the belief that "heartache triggers wisdom." He also described superstitions regarding "praying for my own healing because it may not be God's intention for me."

The second session was conducted approximately 6 weeks after diagnosis. At the second session, this patient listed as intervening losses: "My voice changed. I left my girlfriend, and then my new girlfriend left me." At that time, the grief inventory revealed a predominance of endorsed items in the domain of affect. For the first time, the guilt item was endorsed; and sleep disturbance and social withdrawal were described. His coping repertoire at that time included walks, distraction, "setting priorities," and prayer.

The art task included a self-portrait which consisted of a realistic full-face drawing (Fig 17-18). The crown of the head was closed. Facial asymmetry was noted. Specifically, the right face was passive, and the

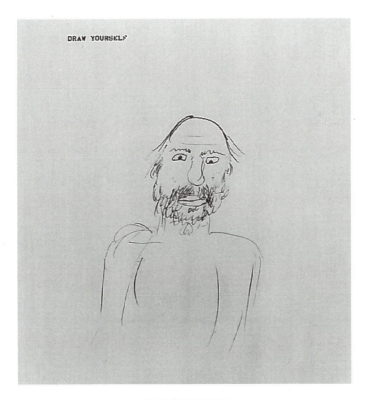

FIGURE 17-18

shoulder was undefined with motion artifact in the up/down direction. The left shoulder was level and broad. No thorax or lower body was drawn in the picture, and the arms were incomplete. The voice drawing task produced a geometric pattern of ovals, triangles, half-ellipses, and shaft-shaped rectangles (Fig 17-19). A line underscores this figure, and superimposed on it is a waveform which consists of smoothly undulating and sharply peaked upward protuberances. Only the midsection of this waveform touches the baseline.

The third session occurred 15 months after the patient's initial diagnosis. At that point, he felt that the prognosis for full return of his voice

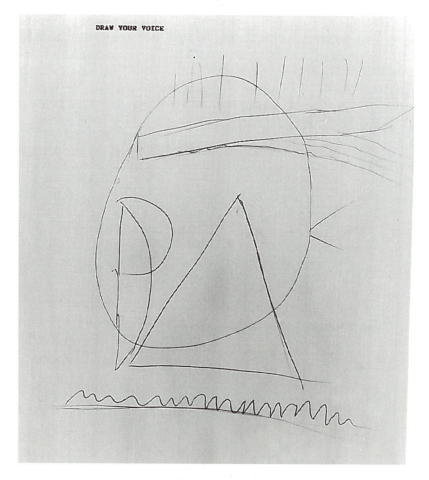

FIGURE 17-19

was "not great." There had been some intervening losses, including loss of illusions about his career, loss of significant relationships, and continued problems from the overuse injury of his wrist which impaired his ability to play the guitar. Items in all four domains of the grief inventory continued to be endorsed. Affect was the most significant, with feelings of sadness and anger, as well as fatigue and helplessness, selected. Interestingly, descriptions of emancipation and relief also were described. Physical sensations continue to include derealization and depersonalization, as well as tightness in the chest and throat. Disbelief, confusion, and preoccupation with the voice were the predominant cognitions. Altered behaviors included sleep disturbance and social withdrawal, as well as restlessness and episodes of crying.

His coping repertoire at that point in his recovery included praying, relaxation techniques, reading, talking to close friends and parents, exercise, music making, and rationalization, although praying and talking to supportive friends and family were most helpful. He also reported setting aside additional time for himself and slowing down his level of activity as helpful adaptations.

The art from this period included a realistic self-representation done as a pencil sketch (Fig 17-20). In contrast to the previous drawings, it was much less organized. A guitar was prominently figured across the center of the trunk. The right wrist was entirely absent, and the left arm was undeveloped. The lower limbs were replaced with indefinite curved lines. The voice was represented as a vertical rectangle with overlapping lines leaving an opening on the right side (Fig 17-21). A triangle protruded from the midpoint, but did not connect to the upright rectangle. Three obliquely angled lines also extended to the upper righthand corner of the picture. A low-amplitude, jagged waveform also extended across the right-hand midportion of the picture, and a series of short, dashlike lines were obliquely sketched in the lower righthand quadrant. The vector appeared to be downward, although the angle was almost the same as the longer, wavelike lines in the upper righthand quadrant. Another figure resembling a helicopter was suspended at the top of the page in the center. The overall feeling from the picture was that of an abstract tree with a presence hovering overhead.

During the interview, the patient described the effect of his voice injury on his level of physical experience as "having less range and slightly less stamina. My voice cannot project as it used to." His reaction to these effects was described as frustration approximately 1 year prior to the third session. He felt that he had learned to work with and enjoy his voice again. When asked to describe the personal meaning of this experience in his life context, the patient replied, "I saw this as a great loss originally, and I have taken the experience as an opportunity

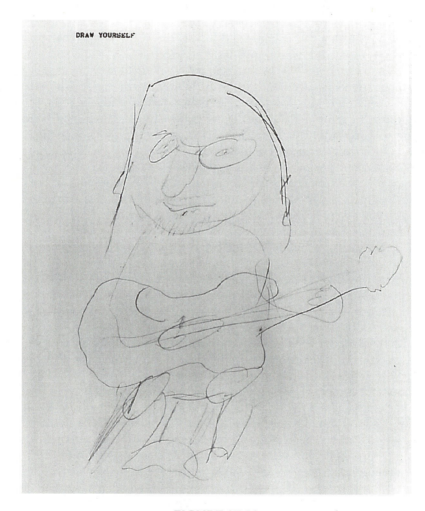

FIGURE 17-20

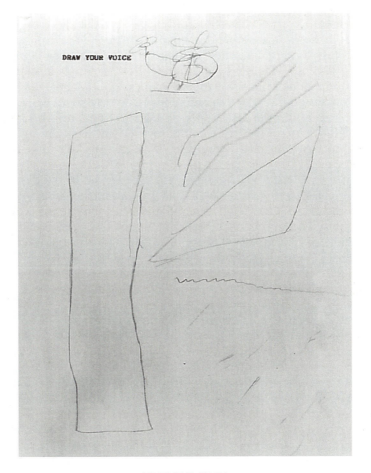

FIGURE 17-21

to rely less on the material world for my happiness and more on the spiritual. This requires discipline." The patient was discharged from treatment, and is actively conducting a professional career as a singer/ songwriter.

Case 7

This patient was a 17-year-old high school senior active in choral singing, as a soloist in various community groups and churches, and also as a flautist. She noted the sudden onset of hoarseness after participation in a strenuous, vocal summer camp. This had been present for approximately 7 months when she was first evaluated at the voice center. On strobovideolaryngoscopic examination, bilateral vocal fold masses due to prior vocal fold hemorrhage were noted. She also had exercise-induced asthma. She met the DSM-IV criteria for clinical depression.

At the first session, this patient endorsed multiple markers in all four domains on the grief inventory, but refused to complete the section for history of prior losses. Her coping repertoire included spending time with numerous peers and a boyfriend, listening to music or playing an instrument, dancing, and having clear, defined goals for herself. On the drawing tasks, her self-portrait was representative and done in color (Plate 17-8). No body was represented below the chest, and the breasts were noticeably absent. The facial expression was one of distrust and sadness in the area of the eyes, and the mouth was in a neutral position. A prominent thrust of the chin is associated with a facial expression of anger. Faint horizontal markings could be seen across the entire neck region. Her drawing of her voice consisted of a cracked and stilled bell (Plate 17-9). She described it as "present internally to herself, but flawed." Golden drops are noted to drip from the clapper of the bell, but the remainder is tarnished. The color utilized to draw the crack is used to define the entire perimeter of the bell itself.

During the interview, the patient described her voice injury in these words, "Self-esteem is defined as your specialness and uniqueness." She recounted that both of her parents were artistically talented, but both gave up their dreams of performance for "steady, responsible jobs." She saw her role as peace-maker between her parents. The patient's mother also appeared depressed, and her relationship with the patient was overinvested and overvigilant regarding the voice and vocal success. The parents were polarized with optimistic and pessimistic views of the potential for the patient's recovery. The patient described herself as "only acceptable and okay when I fill their mold for a satisfactory daughter. They want me to go where they could not."

Session two was conducted approximately 4 months after diagnosis, and the patient had undergone vocal fold surgery for excision of bilateral vocal fold masses. At the second session, she included as losses: "I could not be in the school musical, nor could I be in school concerts, either singing or band." The grief inventory at that time showed a decrease in the choices endorsed in the affective domain with more prominence of the helplessness items. She also endorsed an item about relief. In the physical domain, she continued to describe some dissociative symptoms and throat and chest tightness. Her behavioral choices reflected continued disorganization and disorientation with endorsement of the items regarding sexuality, which is consistent in this phase of grief with a longing for contact. Her cognitions reflected some somatic delusions, but denial was no longer present. Coping responses continued to include positive and supportive friends, reframing her experience to positive aspects, and continued positive self-reinforcement and self-talk. Listening to music which resonated with her emotional experience also was helpful to her.

Art was not fully available at that time because of her refusal to draw a self-portrait. Her drawing of her voice lacked shape definition and consisted of a green circle with an irregular margin, one side flattened, and decentering of the core (Plate 17-10). This was surrounded by a thick layer of brown/black with some elevations of the green core emanating into and reaching through a green outer shell. She described herself as "communication-impaired" and unable to fill her family role as "translator between the parents and as caretaker."

At that time, her parents were very argumentative, and there was significant family stress because her father had lost his job, resulting in financial difficulty. The patient had been told that she could not start college as she had planned and instead needed to work to assist the family. She stated that she was being blamed by her father for a problem related to her tissue healing. At the time of the interview, she was perseverating on any possible behavior in which she might be engaging that could hamper her healing. These were explored, and the negative impact of such self-punitive thoughts was discussed. The rock music she had chosen as most appropriate for pacing her emotions caused her parents to describe her as "different and delinquent." Her grandmother, who had been a constant source of support and acceptance, had died in the intervening period.

Session three was conducted approximately 6 months later. At that point, fat implantation in the vocal folds was planned, but had not yet been performed. The grief inventory responses in the affect domain included descriptions of sadness and anxiety, but some relief. The physical symptoms included a hollow feeling in the abdomen, tightness in the throat and chest, and derealization. The choices in the behavioral domain were those associated with biological depression, chiefly appetite disturbance, sleep disturbance, memory disturbance, concentration disturbance, sadness, and anxiety. In the cognitive domain, she described herself as confused, but auditory delusions of the "lost" voice were no longer present. Coping behaviors included continued positive reframing of the situation, positive self-talk, contact with new friends, playing the piano, and self-acceptance.

The self-portrait this patient produced at the third session (Plate 17-11) was a realistic pencil sketch with the hair done in red magic marker and the eyes a vivid green. The gaze was direct, but despairing. The lips were tightly closed and set in a neutral line. There was no representation below the neck. There was asymmetry in the facial expression which could be seen most readily by masking first one, then the other side of the paper. The right side of the face had less tone, and the facial expression, especially surrounding the eyes, was extremely sad. Although ears had been included in the drawing on both sides, the right ear was incomplete. The left side of the face has less sadness in the area of the eye and slightly more definition to the musculature of the face. The left ear is somewhat prominent and appears to be protruding through the strands of red hair. In the drawing of the voice, a three-dimensional cube with an opening is portrayed with three round balls colored pink, blue, and orange (Plate 17-12). This is accompanied by a caption which reads, "This is a box with balls that had spilled out. To me, this is my voice. It has the potential and the materials to be full, it just needs help to complete it."

During the interview, the patient noted that, "My voice is adding tension to the tension in my parents' marriage." The consequence of her injury and its treatment brought her to the voice center and exposed her to city life and to the local arts community. The patient reported that she felt increasingly more comfortable with her own identity, but that her parents were "afraid of my negative transformation and afraid I'll leave them." She contrasted the effects on her voice of the stress level at home with a period of time during which she travelled to Europe with a performance group. According to the patient, her support system was disintegrating, and all of her friends were leaving for college. For the very first time, she described feeling frightened about the upcoming surgery. "I am tense and drifting." The patient had a successful fat implantation and an uneventful postoperative period. She continued in voice therapy and demonstrated slow, steady improvement in vocal quality.

DISCUSSION

The patients described in this chapter were participants in a research project designed to identify coping responses after perceived voice loss. The methodology offered a variety of means for assessing those responses. The art tasks allowed another window on the experiential world of these "communication-impaired" performers which was more valuable than initially expected. Their voices spoke eloquently in their writing, honest endorsement of inventory items reflecting their personal pain, quotations, and drawings.

Participants were asked to describe and explain their artwork at each session. The psychotherapist refrained from interpreting during the session, but used the drawings to direct the interview toward conflicts or somatic foci symbolized in the art. The research design did not include evaluation of treatment approaches, and these patients did not engage in psychotherapy with the author. However, coping appeared to improve in these patients as a result of their participation, which offered them the opportunity for self-reflection and description of their experiences.

CONCLUSION

The cases presented from this very preliminary research were included to permit observation rather than statistical conclusion. The number of subjects in the study to date is too small to offer valid statistical inference. Nevertheless, the psychological professional familiar with grief counseling and grief therapy will recognize characteristic features. The psychological professional interested in medical psychology in general, and arts medicine psychology specifically, should view the period after vocal injury in professional voice users as appropriate for preventative psychological intervention and should take responsibility for facilitating the tasks of mourning and monitoring mental status for clinically significant changes. He or she can facilitate the process by recognizing promptly unacceptable, split-off responses or the failure to move through any particular response, and by applying therapeutic interventions, including guided drawing assignments, to help the patient journey toward healthy adaptation. Education of colleagues about the normalcy of such responses and the availability and efficacy of supportive psychotherapy permits patients to be referred promptly and offered appropriate treatment.

REFERENCES

1. Janosik E. *Crisis Counseling: A Contemporary Approach*. Boston, MA: Jones and Bartlett Publishing Inc; 1986:3-19.
2. Lindemann E. The symptomatology and management of acute grief. *Am J Psychiatry*. 1944;101:141-149.
3. Bowlby J. *Attachment and Loss: Loss, Sadness, and Depression*. New York, NY: Basic Books; 1980;3:9.
4. Worden JW. *Grief Counselling and Grief Therapy: A Handbook for the Mental Health Practitioner*. New York, NY: Springer Publishing Company; 1982:19-33.
5. Rando T. *Grief, Dying, and Death: Clinical Interventions for Care-Givers*. New York, NY: Research Press; 1984:48-56.
6. Kübler-Ross E. In: Furth G, ed. *The Secret World of Drawings: Healing Through Art*. Boston, Mass: Sigo Press; 1988.

7. Kübler-Ross E. *Living with Death and Dying.* New York, NY: Macmillan Books; 1981.

8. Kübler-Ross E. *On Death and Dying.* New York, NY: Macmillan Books; 1969.

9. Jung CG. In: Jaffee A, ed. *Memories, Dreams, Reflections.* New York, NY: Pantheon Books; 1963.

10. Bach S. ACTA *Psychosomatica: Spontaneous Paintings of Severely Ill Patients.* Basel, Switzerland: Geigy Press; 1969.

11. Furth G. *The Secret World of Drawings: Healing Through Art.* Boston, Mass: Sigo Press; 1988:34-100.

12. Jacoby J. *The Psychology of C.G. Jung.* London: Routledge and Kegan Paul; 1980:53-54.

13. Anastasi IA. *Psychological Testing,* 6th ed. New York, NY: Macmillan Publishing Company; 1988:594-623.

14. Bolander K. *Assessing Personality Through Tree Drawings.* New York, NY: Basic Books; 1977.

15. Jolles I. *Catalogue for the Qualitative Interpretation of the House, Tree, Person.* Los Angeles, CA: Western Psychological Services; 1971.

APPENDIX

I

Psychological Assessment Instruments

NAME: _____

DATE: _____

HOW MUCH TIME HAS ELAPSED SINCE YOUR DIAGNOSIS AT THIS CENTER?

WHAT VOICE THERAPY AND/OR SURGERY HAVE YOU UNDERGONE TO DATE AT THIS CENTER?

WHAT ADDITIONAL VOICE CARE IS PLANNED?

ACCORDING TO YOUR UNDERSTANDING, WHAT IS THE PROGNOSIS FOR YOUR RETURN TO NORMAL VOICE?

LIFE EVENTS AND RELATIVE STRESS VALUES

USING THIS MODIFICATION OF THE HOLMES AND RAHE SCALE, PLEASE RATE THESE EVENTS FOR THEIR RELATIVE STRESS LEVEL IN YOUR LIFE OVER THE PAST YEAR/PAST SIX (6) WEEKS.

-3 = EXTREMELY NEGATIVE   0 = NEUTRAL   +3 = EXTREMELY POSITIVE

EVENT	RATING SCALE						
	-3	-2	-1	0	+1	+2	+3
DEATH OF PARTNER	-3	-2	-1	0	+1	+2	+3
DIVORCE	-3	-2	-1	0	+1	+2	+3
MARITAL SEPARATION	-3	-2	-1	0	+1	+2	+3
JAIL TERM	-3	-2	-1	0	+1	+2	+3
DEATH OF A CLOSE FAMILY MEMBER	-3	-2	-1	0	+1	+2	+3
PERSONAL INJURY OR ILLNESS	-3	-2	-1	0	+1	+2	+3
MARRIAGE	-3	-2	-1	0	+1	+2	+3
FIRED AT WORK	-3	-2	-1	0	+1	+2	+3
MARITAL RECONCILIATION	-3	-2	-1	0	+1	+2	+3
RETIREMENT	-3	-2	-1	0	+1	+2	+3
CHANGE IN HEALTH OF FAMILY MEMBER	-3	-2	-1	0	+1	+2	+3
PREGNANCY	-3	-2	-1	0	+1	+2	+3
SEX DIFFICULTIES	-3	-2	-1	0	+1	+2	+3
GAIN OF NEW FAMILY MEMBER	-3	-2	-1	0	+1	+2	+3
BUSINESS READJUSTMENT	-3	-2	-1	0	+1	+2	+3
CHANGE IN FINANCIAL STATE	-3	-2	-1	0	+1	+2	+3
DEATH OF A CLOSE FRIEND	-3	-2	-1	0	+1	+2	+3
CHANGE TO DIFFERENT LINE OF WORK	-3	-2	-1	0	+1	+2	+3

	−3	−2	−1	0	+1	+2	+3
CHANGE IN NUMBER OF ARGUMENTS W/ PARTNER	−3	−2	−1	0	+1	+2	+3
MORTGAGE OVER $25,000	−3	−2	−1	0	+1	+2	+3
FORECLOSURE OF MORTGAGE OR LOAN	−3	−2	−1	0	+1	+2	+3
CHANGE IN WORK RESPONSIBILITIES	−3	−2	−1	0	+1	+2	+3
CHILD LEAVING HOME	−3	−2	−1	0	+1	+2	+3
TROUBLE WITH EXTENDED FAMILY	−3	−2	−1	0	+1	+2	+3
OUTSTANDING PERSONAL ACHIEVEMENT	−3	−2	−1	0	+1	+2	+3
PARTNER BEGINS OR STOPS WORK	−3	−2	−1	0	+1	+2	+3
CHANGE IN LIVING CONDITIONS	−3	−2	−1	0	+1	+2	+3
REVISION OF PERSONAL HABITS	−3	−2	−1	0	+1	+2	+3
TROUBLE WITH BOSS	−3	−2	−1	0	+1	+2	+3
CHANGE IN WORK HOURS OR CONDITIONS	−3	−2	−1	0	+1	+2	+3
CHANGE IN RESIDENCE	−3	−2	−1	0	+1	+2	+3
CHANGE IN RECREATION	−3	−2	−1	0	+1	+2	+3
CHANGE IN RELIGIOUS ACTIVITIES	−3	−2	−1	0	+1	+2	+3
CHANGE IN SOCIAL ACTIVITIES	−3	−2	−1	0	+1	+2	+3
CHANGE IN SLEEPING HABITS	−3	−2	−1	0	+1	+2	+3
CHANGE IN EATING HABITS	−3	−2	−1	0	+1	+2	+3
CHANGE IN NUMBER OF FAMILY GET-TOGETHERS	−3	−2	−1	0	+1	+2	+3
CHRISTMAS	−3	−2	−1	0	+1	+2	+3
VACATION	−3	−2	−1	0	+1	+2	+3
MINOR VIOLATIONS OF THE LAW	−3	−2	−1	0	+1	+2	+3
BEGIN A NEW SCHOOL AT HIGHER ACADEMIC LEVEL	−3	−2	−1	0	+1	+2	+3
DROPPING A COURSE	−3	−2	−1	0	+1	+2	+3
FINANCIAL DIFFICULTY WITH TUITION	−3	−2	−1	0	+1	+2	+3
FAILING AN IMPORTANT EXAM	−3	−2	−1	0	+1	+2	+3
CHANGING A MAJOR	−3	−2	−1	0	+1	+2	+3
CHANGING SCHOOLS	−3	−2	−1	0	+1	+2	+3

STRESS MANAGEMENT

FOLLOWING IS A LIST OF STRESS MANAGEMENT STRATEGIES. PLEASE INDICATE HOW OFTEN YOU UTILIZE THIS SKILL FOR EACH ITEM. AT THE END OF THE LIST, SPACE IS PROVIDED TO DESCRIBE OTHER, PERSONAL STRATEGIES.

	SELDOM	SOMETIMES	USUALLY	OFTEN	ALWAYS
I. PERSONAL MANAGEMENT SKILLS: ORGANIZING YOUR TIME					
PLANNING/GOAL SETTING	1	2	3	4	5
MAKING A CLEAR COMMITMENT	1	2	3	4	5
SETTING TIME USE PRIORITIES	1	2	3	4	5
CONTROLLING THE PACE AND TEMPO OF DEMANDS	1	2	3	4	5
II. RELATIONSHIPS: CONTROLLING *YOUR* WORLD					
MAKING FRIENDS	1	2	3	4	5
MAINTAINING CONTACT	1	2	3	4	5
LISTENING TO OTHERS	1	2	3	4	5
ASSERTIVE COMMUNICATION	1	2	3	4	5
STANDING YOUR GROUND (FIGHT)	1	2	3	4	5
LEAVING THE SCENE (FLIGHT)	1	2	3	4	5
TURNING YOUR "SPACE" INTO A HOME	1	2	3	4	5
III. OUTLOOK: CONTROLLING YOUR ATTITUDE					
RELABELING MORE POSITIVELY	1	2	3	4	5
SURRENDERING: "LETTING GO" AND "LETTING BE"	1	2	3	4	5
ACCEPTING YOUR LIMITS	1	2	3	4	5
CREATIVITY AND IMAGINATION	1	2	3	4	5
TALKING TO YOUR SELF KINDLY	1	2	3	4	5
IV. YOUR BODY: BUILDING RESISTANCE AND STAMINA					
EXERCISE	1	2	3	4	5
NUTRITIONAL EATING	1	2	3	4	5
GENTLENESS WITH YOURSELF	1	2	3	4	5
RELAXATION SKILLS	1	2	3	4	5

MY PERSONALIZED COPING SKILLS REPERTOIRE INCLUDES:

_____

_____

MY MOST *EFFECTIVE* COPING SKILLS INCLUDE:

_____

_____

LOSS HISTORY

1. IN ADDITION TO THE LOSSES LISTED ON THE STRESS SCALE, PLEASE DESCRIBE ALL OTHER EVENTS WHICH HAVE BEEN INSTANCES OF LOSS FOR YOU IN THE PAST TWELVE (12) MONTHS/PAST SIX (6) WEEKS.

2. PLEASE DESCRIBE ALL EVENTS WHICH HAVE BEEN INSTANCES OF LOSS FOR YOU OVER THE PAST TEN (10) YEARS.

3. DURING THOSE TIMES OF SIGNIFICANT CHANGE AND/OR LOSS IN YOUR LIFE, WHAT PERSONAL COPING STRATEGIES HAVE BEEN HELPFULLY EFFECTIVE FOR YOU?

PLEASE REVIEW THESE REACTIONS TO A STRESSFUL PERSONAL EVENT. CIRCLE ALL THOSE YOU HAVE EXPERIENCED SINCE THE ON-SET OF YOUR VOICE DISORDER IN THE PRIOR SIX (6) WEEKS.

AFFECT	**PHYSICAL SENSATIONS**
SADNESS	HOLLOWNESS IN ABDOMEN
ANGER	TIGHTNESS IN CHEST
GUILT	TIGHTNESS IN THROAT
SELF-REPROACH	"LUMP" IN THROAT
ANXIETY	OVERSENSITIVITY TO NOISE/LIGHT/MOTION
FATIGUE	FEELING REMOVED FROM THE BODY
HELPLESSNESS	SHORTNESS OF BREATH
SHOCK	FEELING REMOVED FROM REALITY
YEARNING	MUSCLE WEAKNESS
EMANCIPATION	LACK OF ENERGY
RELIEF	MOUTH DRYNESS
NUMBNESS	

BEHAVIORS	**COGNITIONS**
SLEEP DISTURBANCE	DISBELIEF
APPETITE DISTURBANCE	CONFUSION
ABSENT-MINDEDNESS	MEMORY DISTURBANCE
SOCIAL WITHDRAWAL	PREOCCUPATION WITH VOICE
PROMISCUITY	SENSE OF DÉJA VU
DREAMS OF "LOST" VOICE	"HEARING" THE "LOST" VOICE
SIGHING	
SEARCHING FOR CURE	
AVOIDING REMINDERS OF "LOST" VOICE	
RESTLESS OVERACTIVITY	
CRYING	
VISITING PLACES ASSOCIATED WITH "LOST" VOICE	
CARRYING OBJECTS ASSOCIATION WITH "LOST" VOICE	

DRAW YOURSELF

DRAW YOUR VOICE

NAME: _____

DATE: _____ INTERVIEW #: _____

INTERVIEW

I. *MENTAL STATUS EXAMINATION*

  A. *PAST PSYCHIATRIC HISTORY*

  B. *APPEARANCE/PRESENTATION*
    (Grooming, Eye Contact, Psychomotor Activity, Congruence)

  C. *PSYCHOTROPIC MEDICATION*

  D. *DRUG/ALCOHOL PATTERNS*

  E. *SUPPORT SYSTEM*

  F. *ORIENTATION*

  G. *MOOD/AFFECT*

  H. *SUICIDAL/HOMICIDAL FEATURES*

I. *REALITY CONTACT*

J. *THOUGHT PROCESSES/CONTENT*

K. *FUND OF KNOWLEDGE/ABSTRACTION/INSIGHT*

L. *MEMORY*

NAME: _____

DATE: _____   INTERVIEW #: _____

INTERVIEW

II. *EFFECT OF VOCAL INJURY*

    A. WHAT ARE THE EFFECTS ON THE FUNCTION/LEVEL OF PHYSI-CAL EXPERIENCE?

    B. HOW IS THE PATIENT REACTING TO THESE EFFECTS?

    C. WHAT IS THE PERSONAL MEANING OF THE PHYSICAL EXPERI-ENCE IN HIS/HER LIFE CONTEXT?

APPENDIX

Patient History Form for Professional Voice Users

NAME _____ AGE _____ SEX ____ RACE _____

HEIGHT _____ WEIGHT _____ DATE _____

1. How long have you had your present voice problem? _____

   Who noticed it?

   Do you know what caused it? **Yes** ☐ **No** ☐

   If so, what?

   Did it come on slowly or suddenly? **Slowly** ☐ **Suddenly** ☐

   Is it getting: **Worse** ☐ **Better** ☐ or **Same** ☐ ?

2. Which symptoms do you have? **(Please check all that apply)**

   ☐ Hoarseness (coarse or scratchy sound)
   ☐ Fatigue (voice tires or changes quality after speaking for a short period of time)
   ☐ Volume disturbance (trouble speaking) softly ☐ loudly ☐
   ☐ Loss of range (high ☐ , low ☐)
   ☐ Prolonged warm-up time (over 1/2 hr. to warm up voice)
   ☐ Breathiness
   ☐ Tickling or choking sensation while speaking
   ☐ Pain in throat while speaking

☐ Other (Please specify): _____

_____

3. Have you ever had training for your singing voice?
Yes ☐ **No** ☐

4. Have there been periods of months or years without lessons in that time?
Yes ☐ **No** ☐

5. How long have you studied with your present teacher?

Teacher's name: _____

Teacher's address: _____

Teacher's telephone number: _____

6. Please list previous teachers and years during which you studied with them:

7. Have you ever had training for your speaking voice? **Yes** ☐ **No** ☐
If so, list teachers and years of study:

8. In what capacity do you use your voice professionally?

☐ Actor
☐ Announcer (television/radio/sports arena)
☐ Attorney
☐ Clergy
☐ Politician
☐ Salesperson
☐ Teacher
☐ Telephone operator or receptionist
☐ Other (Please specify): _____

9. Do you have an important performance soon? **Yes** ☐ **No** ☐
Date(s): _____

10. Do you do regular voice exercises? **Yes** ☐ **No** ☐
If yes, describe:

11. Do you play a musical instrument?   **Yes** ☐ **No** ☐
    If yes, please check all that apply:

    ☐ Keyboard (Piano, Organ, Harpsichord, Other _____)
    ☐ Violin, Viola
    ☐ Cello
    ☐ Bass
    ☐ Plucked Strings (Guitar, Harp, Other _____)
    ☐ Brass
    ☐ Wind with single reed
    ☐ Wind with double reed
    ☐ Flute, Piccolo
    ☐ Percussion
    ☐ Bagpipe
    ☐ Accordion
    ☐ Other (Please specify): _____

12. Do you warm-up your voice before practice or performance?
    Yes ☐ **No** ☐

    Do you warm-down after using it?   **Yes** ☐ **No** ☐

13. How much are you speaking at present (average hours per day)?
    _____ Rehearsal _____ Performance _____ Other

14. Please check all that apply to you:

    ☐ Voice worse in the morning
    ☐ Voice worse later in the day, after it has been used.
    ☐ Sing performances or rehearsals in the morning
    ☐ Speak extensively (e.g., teacher, clergy, attorney, telephone, work, etc.)
    ☐ Cheerleader
    ☐ Speak extensively backstage or at postperformance parties
    ☐ Choral conductor
    ☐ Frequently clear your throat
    ☐ Frequent sore throat
    ☐ Jaw joint problems
    ☐ Bitter or acid taste; bad breath or hoarseness first thing in the morning
    ☐ Frequent "heartburn" or hiatal hernia
    ☐ Frequent yelling or loud talking
    ☐ Frequent whispering
    ☐ Chronic fatigue (insomnia)
    ☐ Work around extreme dryness
    ☐ Frequent exercise (weight lifting, aerobics, etc.)
    ☐ Frequently thirsty, dehydrated
    ☐ Hoarseness first thing in the morning
    ☐ Chest cough
    ☐ Eat late at night

☐ Ever used antacids
☐ Under particular stress at present (personal or professional)
☐ Frequent bad breath
☐ Live, work, or perform around smoke or fumes
☐ Traveled recently: When: _____
☐ Where: _____

15. Your family doctor's name, address and telephone number:

16. Your laryngologist's name, address and telephone number:

17. Recent cold? **Yes** ☐ **No** ☐

18. Current cold? **Yes** ☐ **No** ☐

19. Have you been evaluated by an allergist? **Yes** ☐ **No** ☐
    If yes what allergies do you have:
    [none, dust, mold, trees, cats, dog, foods, other: _____ **]**
    (Medication allergies are covered elsewhere in this history form.)
    If yes, give name and address of allergist:

20. How many packs of cigarettes do you smoke per day?
    Smoking history
    ☐ Never
    ☐ Quit. When? _____
    ☐ Smoked about _____ packs per day for _____ years.
    ☐ Smoke _____ packs per day. Have smoked for _____ years.

21. Do you work in a smoky environment? **Yes** ☐ **No** ☐

22. How much alcohol do you drink? **[none, rarely, a few times per week, daily]** If daily, or few times per week, on the average, how much do you consume? **[1, 2, 3, 4, 5, 6, 7, 8, 9, 10, more]** glasses per **[day, week]** of **[beer, wine, liquor]**
    Did you used to drink more heavily? **Yes** ☐ **No** ☐

23. How many cups of coffee, tea, cola, or other caffeine-containing drinks do you drink per day? _____

24. List other recreational drugs you use **[marijuana, cocaine, amphetamines, barbiturates, heroin, other** _____ **]**

25. Have you noticed any of the following? **(Check all that apply)**

☐ Hypersensitivity to heat or cold
☐ Excessive sweating
☐ Change in weight: gained/lost _____ lbs. in _____ weeks/ _____ months
☐ Change in your voice
☐ Change in skin or hair
☐ Palpitation (fluttering) of the heart
☐ Emotional lability (swings of mood)
☐ Double vision
☐ Numbness of the face or extremities
☐ Tingling around the mouth or face
☐ Blurred vision or blindness
☐ Weakness or paralysis of the face
☐ Clumsiness in arms or legs
☐ Confusion or loss of consciousness
☐ Difficulty with speech
☐ Difficulty with swallowing
☐ Seizure (epileptic fit)
☐ Pain in the neck or shoulder
☐ Shaking or tremors
☐ Memory change
☐ Personality change

For females:

Are you pregnant?   **Yes** ☐ **No** ☐
Are your menstrual periods regular?   **Yes** ☐ **No** ☐
Have you undergone hysterectomy?   **Yes** ☐ **No** ☐
Were your ovaries removed?   **Yes** ☐ **No** ☐
At what age did you reach puberty?
Have you gone through menopause?   **Yes** ☐ **No** ☐

26. Have you ever consulted a psychologist or psychiatrist? **Yes** ☐ **No** ☐
Are you currently under treatment? **Yes** ☐ **No** ☐

27. Have you injured your head or neck (whiplash, etc.)? **Yes** ☐ **No** ☐

28. Describe any serious accidents related to this visit.
None _____

29. Are you involved in legal action involving problems with your voice?
Yes ☐ **No** ☐

30. List names of spouse and children:

31. Brief summary of ENT problems, some of which may not be related to your present complaint.

☐ Hearing loss   ☐ Ear pain
☐ Ear noises   ☐ Facial pain
☐ Dizziness   ☐ Stiff neck
☐ Facial paralysis   ☐ Lump in neck
☐ Nasal obstruction   ☐ Lump in face or head
☐ Nasal deformity   ☐ Trouble swallowing
☐ Nose bleeds   ☐ Trouble breathing
☐ Mouth sores   ☐ Excess eye skin
☐ Excess facial skin   ☐ Eye problem
☐ Jaw joint problem
☐ Other (Please specify): _____

32. Do you have or have you ever had:

☐ Diabetes   ☐ Seizures
☐ Hypoglycemia   ☐ Psychological therapy or counseling
☐ Thyroid problems   ☐ Frequent bad headaches
☐ Syphilis   ☐ Ulcers
☐ Gonorrhea   ☐ Kidney disease
☐ Herpes   ☐ Urinary problems
☐ Cold sores (fever blisters)   ☐ Arthritis or skeletal problems
☐ High blood pressure   ☐ Cleft palate
☐ Severe low blood pressure   ☐ Asthma
☐ Intravenous antibiotics   ☐ Lung or breathing problems
    or diuretics   ☐ Lung or breathing problems
☐ Heart attack   ☐ Unexplained weight loss
☐ Angina   ☐ Cancer of (_____)
☐ Irregular heartbeat   ☐ Other tumor (_____)
☐ Other heart problems   ☐ Blood transfusions
☐ Rheumatic fever   ☐ Hepatitis
☐ Tuberculosis   ☐ AIDS
☐ Glaucoma   ☐ Meningitis
☐ Multiple sclerosis
☐ Other illnesses (Please specify): _____

33. Do any blood relatives have:

☐ Diabetes   ☐ Cancer
☐ Hypoglycemia   ☐ Heart disease
☐ Other major medical problems such as those above.
☐ Please specify: _____

34. Describe serious accidents unless directly related to your doctor's visit here.

    ☐ None
    ☐ Occurred with head injury, loss of consciousness, or whiplash
    ☐ Occurred without head injury, loss of consciousness, or whiplash
    ☐ Describe:

35. List all current medications and doses (include birth control pills and vitamins).

36. Medication allergies

    ☐ None   ☐ Novocaine
    ☐ Penicillin   ☐ Iodine
    ☐ Sulfa   ☐ Codeine
    ☐ Tetracycline   ☐ Adhesive tape
    ☐ Erythromycin   ☐ Aspirin
    ☐ Keflex/Ceclor/Ceftin   ☐ X-ray dyes
    ☐ Other (Please specify): _____

37. List operations:

    ☐ Tonsillectomy (age _____)   ☐ Adenoidectomy (age _____)
    ☐ Appendectomy (age _____)   ☐ Heart surgery (age _____)
    ☐ Other (Please specify): _____

38. List toxic drugs or chemicals to which you have been exposed:

    ☐ Streptomycin, Neomycin, Kanamycin   ☐ Lead
    ☐ Other. Please list: ☐ Mercury

39. Have you had x-ray *treatments* to your head or neck (including treatments for acne or ear problems as a child), treatments for cancer, etc.?
    Yes ☐   **No** ☐

40. Describe serious health problems of your spouse or children.

    ☐ None

INDEX

X

Y

Z